Black Men, Intergenerational Colonialism, and Behavioral Health

Donald E. Grant Jr.

Black Men, Intergenerational Colonialism, and Behavioral Health

A Noose Across Nations

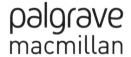

Donald E. Grant Jr.
Mindful Training Solutions
Los Angeles, CA, USA

Pacific Oaks College
Pasadena, CA, USA

ISBN 978-3-030-21113-4   ISBN 978-3-030-21114-1   (eBook)
https://doi.org/10.1007/978-3-030-21114-1

This Palgrave Macmillan imprint is published by the registered company Springer Nature Switzerland AG.
The registered company address is: Gewerbestrasse 11, 6330 Cham, Switzerland

This book is dedicated to my son, my brother, my father, my grandfather, my uncles, my god sons, my fraternity brothers and every other Black man in the world who has ever been told explicitly or implicitly that he is anything less than a King.

PREFACE

The experiences that occur across one's lifespan shape them in ways that often remain elusive until the luxury of reflection arises. In spite of our awareness, or lack thereof, these experiences imprint our personhood in very predictable ways. It wasn't until I was an adult, had lived away from home for a decade and traveled the world that I began to see the imprints of my experiences on my life. It would be in subsequent decades that I would begin to understand them, the ways they intertwined with one another and the varied ways they manifested themselves in my world and in the worlds of others.

"*1989, the number, another summer. Sound of the funky drummer. Music hitting your heart 'cause I know you got soul*" Public Enemy screamed into my eighth grade ears. They continued, "*What we need is awareness, we can't get careless. You say what is this? My beloved let's get down to business. Mental self-defensive fitness.*" That same year, five teenagers—all boys of color—were charged with the assault and rape of a female jogger in New York's Central Park. They would later become known as The Central Park Five. The boys were all convicted (in two separate trials) and jailed in 1990 even after DNA evidence from the rape kit confirmed their lack of involvement. In 1992, Spike Lee released *Malcom X*, an autobiographical sketch portraying the life of the noted civil rights leader. I was a freshman at City Honors High School, a diverse honors magnet school on the east-side of Buffalo, NY. Buffalo's eastside, where I also grew up, is a historic community where many Black people were shrouded in safety along the Underground Railroad and where their children raised their children after

The Great Migration. I wore my Malcolm X medallion and was unapologetically proud of my blackness.

I was a rising senior at Hampton University the summer of 1998 when James Byrd Jr. was murdered by three White supremacists in Jasper Texas. Byrd was still alive as his murderers dragged his body along an asphalt road for three miles. I can still remember feeling my naivety's naivety melting from my body as I learned the details of his murder. By this time, I had seen *Do the Right Thing* and *Boyz in the Hood*; hell, I was a boy in the hood. I had read James Baldwin, Alice Walker, August Wilson and Cornell West. I could reflect on my feelings as I touched former plantations during my family's annual Spring trip to Shelby, North Carolina. Even with all this, Byrd's lynching was something new to accommodate into my recently adulted brain.

I was ending my second year as a Baltimore City Public School science teacher during the summer of 2002 when HBO released its smash hit *The Wire*, which was also set in Baltimore. That same year, the sentences of The Central Park Five were commuted after an incarcerated murderer and serial rapist confessed and provided corroborating DNA evidence. I was working with underserved kids, in an over-extended city that ran an under-resourced school district. I knew about injustice, racism and discrimination. What I didn't know was the depth with which these things lived in the stories of our souls.

As I traveled the world I learned that my unique experience was less unique than I thought. Sure, almost all Black men experience racism and discrimination. I knew that. What I didn't know was the scope, depth and deliberateness of the sustainable models created to impact contemporary Black men and boys in every generation across every continent where they live. I have sat with Black men in their hometowns from Paris to London and Brighton. I have broken bread with brothers from Melbourne to Toronto and Florence. I drank whiskey with Black men in their local bars in Cape Town and Malaga. Me and these men shared a common experience. A visceral one that results in a proverbial head nod familiar to us all. When our spoken languages of origin failed to translate directly, our souls' experiences seemed to share a common lexicon. Each of us had experienced development in a geographic space that had been deliberately structured to maintain our oppression and separation, a fact that many of us were left blind to for decades. A hidden and insidiously veiled agenda that effectively cloaks the ways in which the ecological experiences across our lifespans impact who we are to become.

After I left the classroom, I practiced as a clinical psychologist for the Los Angeles County Department of Mental Health. It would be here that I would truly see the synergistic systems of disenfranchisement at play; it forced a reflection of my own. I began to remember the intergenerational nature of poverty, substance abuse and school attrition I saw in my community as a kid. Here I was, an adult, living thousands of miles away from where I was born but seeing the same thing, years later. There was something to this code that required breaking, something that would come in the following 2014 email:

> Good Afternoon Dr. Grant,
>
> I do not know if you remember me … I was one of your students back when you were a science teacher … I just wanted to contact you to say thank you. You may not remember but you had a talk with me right after I failed your final exam. You spoke with me about seeing my potential and told me that everything in life had to be earned. I consider that conversation I had with you that day one of the defining moments of my life. Even though you gave me some leeway (thankfully) with my grade, I assure you the talk you had with me that day was not in vain.

He goes on to describe his academic successes, work as an engineer in Washington DC and grad school plans. He closes his spontaneous correspondence with:

> I just wanted to let you know that everything I have done and will do educationally and professionally is all because of a science teacher who did not want to see another young black youth squander an opportunity. Thank you again Dr. Grant and I wish you nothing but all the best.

It is for this young Black man and all the other Black men and boys, even those yet to be conceived, that this book is purposed. Each Black baby boy born into nations dominated by Eurocentric norms is imprinted with experiences created to harm. Each adult who comes into contact with Black boys must understand the interconnectedness of history's influence on Black male development. Clinicians, politicians, educators, medical doctors, therapists, case managers, researchers, attorneys, police officers, judges and coaches all need to understand the magnitude of force that lives at the intersection of the Black male ethno-gender identity.

A vast set of events, experiences and activities litter the development of people across the entire duration of their life. After decades, nature versus nurture discussions and their varied iterations continue to surface among research circles. Scientists and clinicians spend hours in laboratories, communities and clinics attempting to identify the most significant factors affecting outcomes in the lives of individuals and the varied spaces in which they develop. These risk and protective factors are often disproportionately distributed among clearly demarcated demographic groups throughout the world. They are also associated with meaningful outcomes for these groups. Globally, women exist inside a set of systems that support misogyny and male privilege, while children—our most vulnerable asset—develop in systems that present daily life and death consequences. Each of these experiences requires deliberately unique ecological scaffolding to enhance protective factors that increase safety and promote positive outcomes for each of the respective groups.

It is my hope that students will use this book to become practitioners dedicated to imbuing their practices with cultural empathy, that parents will be inspired to fill their homes with welcoming symbols of respite for the Black men and boys returning home injured each evening, that adjudicating bodies will be moved to resist the practices that allow Black men and boys to languish as monetized stock, that child welfare systems prioritize the employment of tools to ensure that Black boys find forever parents that understand their experience, and finally that Black men and boys across the diaspora fight against the divisions presented to us as our own.

Los Angeles, CA   Donald E. Grant Jr.

About the Book

Eurocentrism is built from a viewpoint and knowledge-producing methodology that narrowly defines our current model of global power. This perspective took hold centuries ago in varied European countries and resulted in a hegemony and epistemology that define behavioral norms, beauty standards, rubrics of academic success and psychological thresholds of wellness. Europe and North America are the continental homes of many countries where White members of European descent both hold the status of population majority and are tasked with (intentionally or not) operationalizing Eurocentrism and all the dominant cultural norms that accompany it. In addition to the dominant culture citizenry of these nations, many countries are also home to a notable number of individuals who are neither White nor of European descent. Individuals and families of Asian, Latin, Arab and African descent have called these nations home for generations. Their intergenerational and individual development across time has taken place on continents dominated by Eurocentric frameworks of power and in countries where success is measured with Euronormative yard-sticks.

Men and boys of African descent who live in countries that have a history of colonialism, have actively enslaved Africans and who ascribe to a dominant White national context experience a unique set of ecological risks with significant consequences for their socio-cultural trajectories across most all domains. This interface creates livelihoods that uniquely position Black boys developing in nations dominated by White cultural norms in severe danger.

Terms like historical, transgenerational, intergenerational and collective trauma have all been used interchangeably throughout research to describe how different groups of people share collective experiences across generations that have a significant bearing on their development. In this work, the terms are used interchangeably to honor the nomenclature applied in the literature and studies cited. Although they are not all synonymous, they share an important underlying spirit which illustrates how the experiences of one's ancestors influence current systems and the individuals in them in a very real way.

Meta-analyses demonstrate that men of African descent in certain nations across the diaspora experience outcomes that rarely match those of their dominant culture male counterparts. This is particularly true where citizens of White European descent set standards for dominant culture norms. The etiologies and epidemiology of these socio-cultural concerns are varied and complex. Existences grounded in these historical contexts result in dangerously powerful ecosystems. The experiences of Black men and boys in these nations are heavily impacted by life-altering events uniquely common to them. Psychosocial, socio-cultural and behavioral health data for Black men in four industrialized nations were assessed across domains including but not limited to employment, academic attainment, adjudication, trauma exposure, substance abuse and somatic illness. The USA, France, the UK and Canada each have general populations of over 30 million people, a dominant culture of White European descent and specific municipalities where at least 5% of the population is of African descent.

The goals of this study, some of which have yet to be seen, are many and vast. For some, the analysis will increase understanding of how certain factors work together to the collective global detriment of Black men and boys. For some, it will highlight the strength-based strategies, required efforts and available opportunities to optimize positive outcomes. For others, it will provide a shared global context whereby your experience and history are validated as a part of a collective in a way that engenders strength, resilience and post-traumatic growth.

Africa is often described and researched as an expansive country instead of a continent housing many diverse countries. As a result, the universality of negative stereotypes about it grows wildly and widely unchallenged. While in Canada, one might say "Parts of Toronto are unsafe", but you would rarely hear "North America (or even Canada) is unsafe". This is because in each North American country, the states and provinces are identified at best by county and at worst by region (northeast, southwest). Due to the historical context of this study, deliberate efforts were made to not support those flawed and damaging paradigms. This text measuredly juxtaposes geographic regions on the continent to specific chronosystems throughout history. In doing so, a clear illustration is made of the depth and value of Africa's history and its pre-colonial existence.

Chapter 1: *Noble Nooses* provides a framework that grounds the study in a historical context of origin, strength and resilience often subject to negationism. The singular view of the continent of Africa is challenged through the multi-disciplinary exploration of both pre-historic and pre-colonial Africa. Using paleoarchaeological and anthropological research, this chapter covers several millennia to describe the ways in which the earth was populated (Out of Africa I), the spaces where the original anatomically modern humans resided and with whom they interbred (Out of Africa II), which ethno-linguistic families thrived in which geographical regions (Bantu Migration) and the strengths in the pre-historic migratory patterns resulting in the structure of Ancient Africa. The second half of the chapter highlights the pre-colonial regal histories across the continent. Exploring the Black Pharaohs of the 25th Dynasty, Taharqa's deliverance of Hezekiah, the Ghanaians, the Kushites and many more provides evidence of spaces to engender resilience in youth and hold content for anti-bias tool development. The chapter ends by building connections between contemporary (Malcolm X) and historical (Shaka Zulu) Black men across the diaspora.

Chapter 2: *Birth of a Noose* explores and analyzes the intracontinental aspects of thirteenth-, fourteenth- and fifteenth-century Europe. Countries who had a hand in the Transatlantic Slave Trade, European imperialism and African colonialism are investigated alongside a model of nationalistic development supporting the context that led to each country's individual participation in the implementation, maintenance and eventual dismantling of the Transatlantic Slave Trade. Portugal, Spain (Castile), England and France are explored through a developmental lens using events like The Hundred Years War, The Peasants' Revolt, The Bubonic Plague, The War of the Roses and The Age of Discovery as events that informed their nationalism and supported their imperialistic lust. The chapter closes with the development of a global economic system that demonstrates how European players managed to birth the system of enslavement based on bio-genetic features including skin color, perception of savagery and specific disease immunity resulting in an African preference.

Chapter 3: *Cross-Continental Nooses* details the intricate involvement of Portugal, Spain, England and France in the Transatlantic Slave Trade and the acute factors of success which include trade monopolies and ascientos (Papal Bulls), exploration charters (Royal Africa Company), investors (Charles II, John Locke) and insurers. The history of the cotton plant, the European Industrial Revolution and the Liberation of Haiti are implicated as catalyzing factors driving American slavery to exponential growth and cruelty. The chapter moves into the American Civil War by first exploring American land expansion (Louisiana Purchase), exponential population growth and the end of the Lancashire Cottage Industry. The chapter closes with an exploration of the histories of contemporary businesses like Lehman Brothers, Lloyds of London, Aetna Insurance, Barclays and JP Morgan Chase. Narratives and litigation records show how these organizations monetized the African slave trade to leverage resources for the building of their personal empires and global brands.

Chapter 4: *Scientific Nooses* details the theoretical constructs of the text to create an evidence base of theory on which the reader will ground the history presented. Intergenerational (Historic) Trauma, the Bio-Ecological Model of Development, Blumenbach's Theory and Epigenetics are just some of the concepts explored. These theories are explored through historic decisions, programs, policies and documents. Political violence and the Rwandan Genocide are used to explain the transmission of trauma via different theoretical frameworks (psychodynamic, family systems), models (socio-cultural) and biological mechanisms like epigenetics (methylation, histone modification and chromatin remodeling). The chapter closes with the contemporary oppressive forces that Black men experience in Euronormative nations from racist "Bamboula" cookies to political exclusion and the organizations created in these nations to address racism.

Chapter 5: *Post-Traumatic Nooses* is an in-depth exploration into the ways in which the most prominent aspects of historically oppressive models reinvented themselves across chronosystems and generations. Comparisons between nineteenth-century programs like convict leasing and debt peonage and twenty-first-century practices like bail/bond structures and predatory pay day loan practices show similarities demonstrative of a possible relationship. When juxtaposed to the history of litigation, psychological testing, federal and private experimentation, eugenics, mass incarceration and institutionalized racism, the maintenance of post-colonial oppression across time is illustrated. Black male vilification across media—print, theatrical, audio, video and digital—is identified and illustrated as a significantly complicit structure for oppression's continuity against Black men and boys. A relationship is established between the aforementioned and contemporary research on employment, academic attainment, adjudication, somatic and mental illnesses, trauma exposure, substance abuse and the stories of Black men and boys across the diaspora who have died during or immediately following engagement with police, security and/or law enforcement.

Chapter 6: *Noose Knots* identifies and illustrates the risk and protective factors in the contemporary ecological systems of each nation (USA, UK, France and Canada). This chapter assesses the current behavioral health and mental wellness outcome data (special education, substance abuse, exposure to trauma, employment rates, school attrition rates, incarceration rates, etc.) and links them to ecological risk factors generated by each nation's participation in the Transatlantic Slave Trade and the colonization of Africa and other territories. An exploration of psychological phenomena associated with oppressive forces (learned helplessness, stereotype threat, disidentification, self-fulfilling prophecy, racial stress, stigma, bias and access) contextualizes the data presented. This chapter ends by connecting the risk and protective factors to the statistical outcomes illustrated in biological and ecological markers (hair cortisol concentrations, cancer, diabetes, leading causes of death) along with an exploration of the dangers associated with frequent misdiagnoses (ASD, ODD, ADHD, IED and CD) and the etiological practices behind them.

Chapter 7: *Healing Noose Scars* is grounded in resiliency theory, ecological restructuring, mindfulness, collectivistic principles and Afrocentric psychological paradigms (Collective Coping, Racism Trauma) and tools (Africultural Coping Systems Inventory, Racism-Related Coping Scale). Strategies that will enhance Black male relationships across the diaspora to promote a more cohesive and connected view of the Black male experience as it develops inside of the Euronormative narrative are discussed. Recommendations are made on teacher training, socio-emotional learning development, anti-bias curriculum implementation, faith-based interventions, historically Black college and university (HBCU) support, recruitment and retention of Black male educators, and the addition of culturally empathic services at predominantly White institutions (PWIs).

CONTENTS

About the Author

Donald E. Grant Jr., PsyD began his career as a middle school science teacher in Baltimore, MD, after graduating from Hampton University with a Bachelor's degree in Biology. Having grown up in an under-resourced Buffalo, NY, community, he knew very quickly that the kids he was teaching needed more than he had to offer at the time. This prompted Dr. Grant's doctoral studies in Clinical Psychology with an emphasis on Multi-Cultural Community Psychology and a move to Los Angeles, CA, in 2003. His doctoral studies deepened his awareness of systems and their implications, laying the foundation for his research.

Along with his broad work in media, coaching and wellness, Dr. Grant serves as Executive Director of the Center for Community and Social Impact at Pacific Oaks College in Pasadena, CA. In addition to his prior higher education roles as a clinical training director, core faculty member and academic dean, he has a long history of direct mental health service delivery and administrative oversight for foster care systems and child welfare programs with Los Angeles County Department of Mental Health where he served as a clinical psychologist.

Dr. Grant works diligently to increase awareness on mental wellness issues, parenting, child development and socio-cultural events that impact citizens of our country and our world as an author; an equity, diversity and inclusion trainer and practitioner; an NBC mental health and parenting expert; and a film and documentary consultant through his boutique training and consultation firm, Mindful Training Solutions, LLC.

LIST OF TABLES

CHAPTER 1

Noble Nooses: *Pre-Colonial Kings and the Peopling of the Globe*

Powerful kings and emperors like Piye, Kaleb, Mansa Musa, Masinissa, Taraqa and others lived during a time that feels inconceivably distant on a land many men of African descent have never had the opportunity to visit. Although narratives from the spaces between then and now are riddled with the traumas of enslavement, imperialism and colonialism, they also hold literal and figurative jewels and gems that have been stolen and hidden from plain sight. These duplicitous efforts have been effective at deliberately hiding and strategically dismantling the bridges that connect the men of the past to those of today.

For many people of European descent, there exists a continuous thread of uninterrupted history that bounds populations of different chronosystems together across their entire diaspora. Most White people have a clearly articulated and well-published path by which their collective culture and cultural traditions reached the contemporary times and spaces in which they exist. Even when those histories included traumas like the agriculturally induced mass migrations of the Irish during the Potato Famine, systems aren't aimed at the deliberate erasure of links to the origins of their land and native people. The ancient men of Africa and contemporary men across the diaspora, though separated by time and space, share a socio-culturally grounded genetic continuity that has been deliberately censured and censored. These efforts inoculate the processes associated with individual and collective efforts to disassemble the history of oppression and its contemporary systems of disenfranchisement.

© The Author(s) 2019   1
D. E. Grant Jr., *Black Men, Intergenerational Colonialism, and Behavioral Health*, https://doi.org/10.1007/978-3-030-21114-1_1

The African continent and its progeny hold the keys to a collective history that would have undoubtedly amalgamated to operational prominence absent systems of structured oppression and anti-Black supremacy. The paleontological and archaeological records of the continent and its people demonstrate longevity, innovation, resilience, collectivism, resistance and courage. The many men responsible for these archaic achievements across their ethno-linguistic spheres are the forefathers to the entire diaspora of Black men across the world. The chronological and geographic distances between contemporary Black men and these Black men of antiquity created great opportunities for negationists, revisionists, neo-Nazis and White supremacist to effectively co-opt their narratives to the devices of oppression.

THE DELIVERANCE

In 2019, *Parts of the Holy Bible, selected for the use of Negro Slaves, in the British West-Indian Islands* (1807) was made part of an exhibit at the Museum of the Bible in Washington, D.C. A standard Christian Bible includes 1189 chapters, but this one consists of only 232. The redacted Bible was on loan to the museum from Fisk University, a Historically Black College/University (HBCU) in Nashville, TN. One of only three known copies in the world (the other two are on display at universities in Britain), the majority of the Old Testament is totally absent, as is half of the New Testament. The Bibles were printed by the Missionary Society for the Conversion of Negro Slaves and used to convert enslaved people to Christianity (Martin, 2018).

The Hebrew Bible often referred to as the Old Testament of the Christian Bible represents a collection of writings compiled and preserved that chronicle Jewish history and genealogy. Propagandized Bibles are not unique; this is only one aspect of the evidence demonstrating how Christianity was used to both convert the souls of the enslaved while simultaneously oppressing them. This Bible and others like it were edited with the deliberate omission of chapters and verses thought to potentially insight self-esteem among the enslaved and rebellion against the enslavers. Verses that supported justice and liberation were removed. Verses that reinforced subservience and compliance were retained. In addition to raising faith and imbuing hopeful joy or coercing a set of behavioral norms, this religious text, like many others, has been used and weaponized to fashion stories that maintain disparities resulting in generations of suffering and despair.

The continent of Africa has experienced a history that has tattooed her from top to bottom. Many of these tattoos are beautiful works of art that tell stories of love, resilience, innovation, nobility and wealth. The remainder weave themselves up through and around the flesh like the poison of fear from an envenomation, the sting that tells the story of the injustices waged against a land and its people. Since their inception as professional disciplines, the research and literature on anthropology and archaeology have consistently incorporated race and cultural exploration into their work. As a consequence of their longevity, reach across varied sociopolitical contexts and many sub-disciplines, the vast body of work produced is rich and detailed albeit nuanced and at times conflicting. This chapter will ground its focus in the physical and biological paradigms of anthropology and archaeology to explore the histories of the people and cultures of ancient and pre-colonial Africa, their movement across the continent and a shared connectivity to their Black descendants across countries and continents.

Historical negationism is an extreme form of historical revisionism where facts are strategically included or withheld in a deliberate manner to support a new narrative or achieve a new goal. Christianity's ability to manipulate their own Holy text for use as a tool to perpetrate oppression and enslavement is remarkably demonstrative of the oppressive institution's need for a robustly supportive narrative. The manner in which these systems materialized speaks volumes to the weight and value placed upon the institution slavery. While marginalized groups engage historical revisionists to re-incorporate contributions omitted by negationists, people across the globe suffer as the tools of oppression continue to build literal and figurative walls of injury (Etheredge, 2010; Jooste, 2009).

Revered religious texts like the Bible were not immune to such tampering as evidenced by the one on display at the Fisk University Library. This type of negationism as it relates to a religious doctrine is very clear and straightforward. In scenarios less conspicuous than the removal of 80% of an entire book, it might be difficult to determine the deliberateness of this strategy. If this was not done deliberately to disenfranchise, they would have maintained a sense of its integrity and not removed such a large portion. I'm sure any oncological surgeon would agree that the removal of a large tumor from an organ is wrought with many more risks than the removal of a small one. The strategy required to remove a malignant tumor that has taken over 80% of one's GI track requires a team of experts to remove the menacing growth while minimizing assault to the organ system's purposeful functioning. It would be interesting to know how many strategy sessions were held to determine what should remain and what should go. Which verses might inspire or compel enslaved people to see their value and rise to their birthright of freedom against their enslavers?

There are several noteworthy stories illustrated throughout religious text that historians, archaeologists and anthropologists use as points of reference. The deliverance of King Hezekiah and Israel from the Assyrian army is one that is described across three different books of the Bible and celebrated across continents of Christians worldwide. Described in the books of Isaiah, Chronicles and 2nd Kings, the Assyrian siege against Israel was a low point for King Hezekiah and the residents of what would come to be known as The Holy Land. According to the biblical recollection of events, the citizens of Jerusalem were afraid yet prayerful as the Assyrian army grew close and surrounded the walls of the city. Chapter 19 of 2nd Kings focuses on King Hezekiah's handling of the Assyrian siege. His administration was communicating with the Assyrians and continued to receive news of their own demise. Hezekiah and Israel, inspired by the prophet Isaiah, prayed for deliverance. Each verse in this chapter reads as a historical account of communication and engagement—like a court stenographer—yet the end of the chapter tersely transitions into a numinous explanation of events that appear to negate what the historical record supports.

After over 30 verses with descriptions of very tangible and observable activities like exchanging communications, tearing off of clothing, securing prayer garments, praying and consulting elders, the tone for two near-end verses becomes unusually mystified. In chapter 19 of the Bible's 2nd book of Kings, verses 35 and 36 describe the end of the Assyrian siege as follows: "[35]That very night the angel of the LORD went out to the Assyrian camp and killed 185,000 Assyrians troops. When the surviving Assyrians woke up the next morning, they found corpses everywhere. [36]Then King Sennacherib of Assyria broke up his camp and returned to his own land. He went home to his capital of Nineveh and stayed there." The final verse of the chapter describes where, how and by whom King Sennacherib was murdered.

As a part of worldwide curricula, many students learn about the pharaohs of Egypt's antiquity very early on in their academic careers. From the very archaic pharaohs Qa'a and Khufu responsible for the Great pyramid of Giza to the relatively modern pharaohs like Ramses II, Akhenaten and Tutankhamun, this uncontested pharaonic kingdom would rule the area for over 5000 years across over 30 dynasties. Many, however, are sadly—but not surprisingly—unfamiliar with the 25th dynasty of Ancient Egypt that ruled during the eighth century Before Common Era (BCE). For many reasons, negationists have manipulated phenotypic features, topographical maps, narratives and reflections of the country to deliberately separate it geographically, socially and culturally from African continental membership. To be clear, almost all of the pharaohs during the dynastic period of Egypt were Black Africans in spite of attempts from artists, film makers and authors to overtly imbue them with Eurocentric features and sensibilities.

Earlier in 2nd Kings, Chap. 19, verse nine reads: "… King Sennacherib received word that King Taharqa (Taharka) of Ethiopia was leading an army to fight against him." King Taharqa is only mentioned twice in the Bible (again in Chap. 37 of Isaiah) and sparsely throughout the commonly shared record of ancient Egypt. Taharqa, son of Piye, was a noteworthy ruling Pharaoh in Egypt's 25th dynasty, a notably darker-skinned and incidentally less celebrated dynasty than any other. In *The Rescue of Jerusalem: The Alliance between Hebrews and Africans 701BC* (2002), author Henry T. Aubin, Hebrew expert, indicates that the "angel of the LORD" credited with saving King Hezekiah and Jerusalem in 2nd Kings 19:35 was actually a young Taharqa and his army. Aubin and other scholars believe that had Taharqa not intervened on Israel's behalf, this small Hebrew community would have disappeared. Without the survival of Jerusalem, Judaism, a fledgling religion of the time, would not have survived. They add that because Judaism birthed both Christianity and Islam, Taharqa of the 25th Egyptian dynasty would be responsible for the proliferation of each of the three major contemporary world religions.

Unfortunately, in spite of his accomplishments, Taharqa's legacy would largely be painted with the Assyrian rise to power later in the seventh century. This powerful dynasty of darker-skinned kings who revived Egyptian intellectual and artistic roots marked the last pharaohs of the golden age of Egypt. Why is this dynasty of kings noticeably absent from the continent's strategically selected celebratory narratives? Why is this dynasty not as prominently reflected in the Museum of Cairo as others? Why—as late as 2018—might the Sudanese government have supported the plan for the construction of dams to specifically flood miles of Nubian and Kush ruins in Kajba, Shereik and Dal where significant evidence of Black pharaonic history exists (Enough, 2016; Bosshard, 2011)?

In the same way the strategically manipulated Bible of 1807 was used for the conversion of enslaved people to Christianity, less conspicuous efforts have been accepted as rote truths among other truths supported by bodies of evidence. Two significant factors often exacerbate the maintenance of a very rudimentary perspective on which Black cultural history and heritage often rest. First is the insistence that the histories of Black people began only at enslavement and second that the history of the African continent began only when European colonial and imperial entrepreneurs arrived. A true historically grounded understanding of the continent's history requires a collective, strength-based paradigm that honors the origin narrative verified by the archaeological fossil record, uses evidence from anthropological cultural artifacts and tracks the ethnolinguistics phonemic record. Acknowledging the multiplicity of the African people and the nations they created as evidenced by their migration across the continent is critically important to this study. Perhaps most importantly though is the intermingling of details and evidence that tell the stories of power, influence and wealth regarding African nations, all prior to the atrocities of the Transatlantic Slave Trade and European colonial imperialism.

THE SEAT OF ALL CIVILIZATIONS

Commonly held beliefs of racial superiority across the globe seem to dismiss the archaeological record. Even though multi-disciplinary research unequivocally demonstrates that the original members of our human species were African, the behaviors of non-Africans often manifest themselves in paternalistic superiority. The following technical exploration provides an in-depth look at how and where populations migrated, evolved, created communities and differentiated. The history of racial hierarchies and pigmentocracies in our world is antithetical to the fact that most all indigenous people were people of color and descendants of Africans. As early species of ancient man migrated off the continent, modern man had already evolved on the continent. While communities across Africa were advancing in brain size and executive function, Europe was primarily inhabited by proto-humans like Neanderthals and Denisovans. This was until modern humans began their migration (2nd Out of Africa Movement).

Ethno-archaeologists seek to build bodies of research that provide explanations on cultures and their genomic qualities across chronological time, geographical place and esoteric space. Studies of the human genome across the world have had several focal points, and although most are beyond the scope of this work, some exploration is required to ground this research geographically. Exploring research on the human genome to explain the movement of people and their genes across the African continent is important to understanding both the historical depth of Africa's genetic record and the level of diasporic connectedness shared in spite of global geographic displacement (Lemieux, 2018; MacEachern, 2000; McIntosh, 2008; Meyerowitz, 1952).

Africa is the second largest continent on the globe by both geographic size and human population. The land mass itself reaches across both the Northern and Southern Hemispheres, covering over 11 million square miles (Europe 3.9 M mi^2, North America 9.4 M mi^2). Its post-colonial structure is comprised of over 50 unique countries, countless cultures, ethnicities and languages. The continent hosts a myriad of phenotypes from skin tone and hair texture to facial features and height attributions. According to *The History of Geography and Genes* (1994), the "origin of modern humans was in Africa, from which an expansion of the rest of the world started about 100 kiloyears ago (kya)" (Cavalli-Sforza, Menozzi, & Piazza, 1994, p. 154). Most models illustrating the geographic distribution of human genetic attributes focus on the genetic diversity brought to the continent of Africa, but rarely focus on the bi-directional mixing of DNA based on migratory practices of early humans. Early archaeological models explored comparisons of genetic commonalities of modern people in a geographic region to the pre-historic DNA records of people who had inhabited those lands thousands of years before. It wasn't long before researchers realized this was an unreliable methodology based upon a restricted lens. In countries like South Africa, the USA, Canada and Australia, clear evidence demonstrates that the vast majority of current inhabitants are not the genetic, ethnic or cultural descendants of those who occupied those lands prior European colonization.

Modern humans date back about 200 kya and began to migrate to other parts of the world about 100 kya after that. These migrating groups, as might be expected, engaged in gene pool mixing with other pre-historic human groups along their travels. Neanderthals and Denisovans are examples of those archaic groups with whom modern humans would have intermingled and procreated. Researchers fully sequenced the Neanderthal genome in 2010, confirming they and modern humans had engaged in sexual relationships even further back in history than research had initially demonstrated. Fossil records dating back over 40 kya show that although

Denisovans, Neanderthals and modern humans are genetically unique, they not only cohabitated, but procreated together in regions from Siberia to Southeast Asia. "Present day Europeans and Asians have inherited between one and three percent of their DNA from Neanderthals, but Africans have not" (Gibbons, 2016, p. 4). Although the absence of early human DNA in people of African descent is valuable and interesting, the documented inheritance of African DNA by the Altai Neanderthals of Siberia about 100 kya is even more noteworthy (Kuhlwilm & Gronau, 2016). DNA analysis from both within and outside of the continent provides conclusive evidence that Africa hosts greater genetic diversity within its borders when compared to other lands. These analyses also "unambiguously resolved Africans as the deepest single ancestral branch from which all non-African groups arise ..." (Oppenheimer, 2012, p. 770).

The fossil record identifies *Homo heidelbergensis* as the common ancestor to all three of these distinct groups: Anatomically Modern Human (AMH), Neanderthals and Denisovans. *Homo heidelbergensis* was the first early human to live in colder climates, control fire, hunt large animals and build shelters out of wood and stone. Research demonstrates that on at least three distinct historical occasions, the Neanderthals and the Denisovans interbred with what we now know as the modern human. Records of nuclear DNA (nDNA) samples from contemporary European and Asian populations show a clear mix of genetic material from Neanderthals and Denisovans. This is not true for modern Africans, implying that this mix occurred after the "Out of Africa" migration. The Neanderthals and the Denisovans lived in Europe and Asia as early as 250 kya, thousands of years after their evolution. The earliest fossils of archaic humans that were neither Neanderthal nor Denisovan are dated far before this time, begging the question: Where did the Neanderthals and the Denisovan come from and how did they get to Eurasia (Kuhlwilm & Gronau, 2016; Oliver, 2004)?

OUT OF AFRICA MOVEMENTS

Some people argue that modern-day humans never interbred with the archaic humans, but that the genetic overlap was likely due to a common African ancestry that is shared by both the Neanderthal and modern humans. The Serial Founder Effect—a noted theory describing the peopling of the world and how they came to be where they are—features many expansions into new territory by small groups of people. The theory further explains the relationship this phenomenon had on the diversity of genes found in those groups over time. As a result of technological advances and additions to the fossil record, tenets and assumptions based on and informed by the Serial Founders Effect are being questioned and labeled as over-simplified in scope. Archaic humans—ancestors of the Neanderthal—migrated from Africa to Eurasia about a million years ago according to the Out of Africa I theory. *Homo sapiens* evolved between 200 and 300 kya and began their migration from Africa in the Out of Africa II theory model. If this dispersal pattern explanation seems over simplified, it's largely because it is (Pickrell & Reich, 2014).

Research demonstrates that both Out of Africa models occurred over thousands of years, incorporated admixtures of DNA from archaic pre-humans, involved several geographically stratified genetic "bottlenecks" and encompassed at least three different geographic routes off the continent. The first Out of Africa migrations were of pre-historic humans and led to the Eurasian Neanderthal and Denisovan populations. The well-preserved fossil records of these groups are prevalent and have been excavated from lands throughout the Siberian Peninsula and Southeastern Asia. The second Out of Africa migrations were of species within the modern *Homo sapien* phylogenetic branch who traversed the land masses thousands of years later settling in spaces that scientists demonstrate may have still been occupied by pre-historic hominids (Oppenheimer, 2012; Pickrell & Reich, 2014).

Even with such significant progress in archaeological processes, scientific fossil dating techniques, nuclear and mitochondrial DNA mapping analysis and migratory geographic approximation methods, research maintains several ambiguities across a variety of fronts related to the peopling of the globe. Did archaic and modern humans co-exist, and if they did, what happened when they interacted with one another? Under what conditions did both modern and archaic humans migrate from their varied African continental regions? Did either of these groups experience genetic bottlenecks? Did the two groups interbreed with one another, and if they did, were any of their off-spring fertile?

Theories of initial migration point to severe climatic changes that forced both archaic and modern populations of humans from Africa at different times, while others describe an inherent process of migration typical of the world's people. Theories of genetic diversity implicate interbreeding among the three groups that may have led to the absorption of archaic humans into the genetic order of the modern human. Theories on the extinction of archaic humans propose both climatic hypothesis and models that modern humans arrived to the geographies of their archaic ancestors with diseases and infections for which they had no immunity to.

The aforementioned ambiguities are, however, juxtaposed to several incontestable facts held in the detailed and well-documented fossil record of Africa. The oldest fossils of both modern and archaic humans were excavated from regions on the continent of Africa. AMHs migrated out of Africa over 200 kya, and the oldest fossil records of early modern human beings outside the borders of Africa were found at the Misliya caves in Israel and the Jebel Faya archaeological site in the United Arab Emirates. They date back 185 and 125 kya, respectively. Prior to the early twenty-first century, the Omo fossils from the Omo Kibish archaeological site in Ethiopia were thought to be the oldest *Homo sapien* fossils ever excavated. They date back approximately 200 kya. More recent excavations at the Jebel Irhoud site in Morocco unearthed *Homo sapien* fossils and tools that date back 300,000 years. This suggests that modern humans may have not only evolved sooner than we thought, but that they in fact existed more broadly across the continent than evidence originally demonstrated (Oppenheimer, 2012; Pickrell & Reich, 2014).

"Lucy", an *Australopithecus afarensis*, discovered in the 1970s was once the continents' most famous fossil discovery. Although these remains gained great notoriety, their antiquity would pale in comparison to other far more ancient archaeological discoveries. Africa is well known for having the lengthiest record of human existence in the entire world. The world's oldest fossils of AMHs (*H. sapien*) and early evolutionary species of modern humans (*H. erectus*, *H. habilis* and *H. naledi*) were all discovered on the continent of Africa. This unambiguously demonstrates, based on our most contemporary tools of archaeology and science, that the continent of Africa is the seat of civilization and the most likely site of contemporary mans' origin (Kuhlwilm & Gronau, 2016; The National Archives).

Across the continent from the Rising Star cave system in South Africa to Jebel Irhoud in Morocco, fossils of AMHs and others within the same phylogenetic genus have been unearthed. The very first fossil discovery of an archaic AMH on the continent of Africa was made in 1921 by a Swiss miner in Zambia. Its phylogenetic nomenclature became *Homo heidelbergensis*, and it was nicknamed Rhodesian Man. At the time of this publication, the oldest *Homo sapien* fossils discovery had occurred at an archaeological site in Jebel Irhoud, Morocco. Of the remains studied, the mandibular morphology and dental structure were comparable to that of contemporary AMHs. Although the primitive natures of their neurocranial and endocranial morphology demonstrate that their brains were likely smaller and less developed than contemporary man, they are still classified as *Homo sapiens*. Thermoluminescence dating and skeletal morphological analyses of the remains date them back to between 280 and 350 kya (Bower, 2017; Hublin, 2017).

The thirty collective miles of the Olduvai Gorge in the Serengeti Plains of Northern Tanzania hosts fossil deposits dated from over 2 million years ago to as recent as 15 kya, providing one of the most continuous records of human evolution currently known to man. It was here that archaeologist Mary Leaky discovered skull fragments of a hominin, the archaic human *Paranthropus boisei* or OH 5 who was nicknamed "The Nut Cracker" due to the size of its molars. Over 3500 miles away, just outside of Johannesburg are an array of about 15 paleoanthropological sites including: Swartkrans, Sterkfontein and Kromdraai which are collectively referred to as the Cradle of Humankind. To date, more hominid fossils have been unearthed here than any other site in the world (Britannica Olduvai retrieved, 2018a).

Collectively, these archaeologists documented species of early man, their ancestors and their progeny. What is most unique, however, is that all these findings confirm that species like *Homo naledi*, discovered in the Rising Star Cave system also in South Africa, likely existed during the same time period as modern human beings and their direct ancestors (*Homo sapien* and *Homo antecessor*). Although they were more similar to *Homo erectus* and *Homo habilis* than AMHs, they walked the earth at the same time and likely interbred with one another (Hawkins et al., 2017).

A Connected Legacy

What if Black men across the globe were taught very early on that their ancestors were not only the first modern humans to inhabit the earth but that there was connectivity of identity over time? What if parents and teachers were compelled to use—as tool to build foundational self-worth—a timeline that directly connected Black boys to excellence in the ways that other cultural groups do for their boys? Very deliberate efforts have been made to dismantle the shared legacies of greatness that Black men and boys have experienced in spite of unequivocal evidence supported by the historical and archaeological record.

The building of collective links to one another is a critical first step at demonstrating how history exists prior to enslavement and Africa's colonization. The examples of how men are connected through history and genetics are endless. Highlighting them creates a framework to empower young Black men to begin a self-narrative grounded in power, not subordinance. Frantz Fanon, born in 1925 on the French colony of Martinique, was a revolutionary who fought vehemently against colonialism and its impact. His awareness of disparity became a driving force for him after his service for the Free French Forces against the Germans in World War I (WWI) for which he was awarded a Croix de Guerre, the French equivalent to an American Purple Heart. Later, he studied psychiatry in Lyon where he would be influenced by the writings of French philosopher and political activist Jean-Paul Sartre. As a psychiatrist he analyzed the psychological effects of colonial oppression on Black people in his 1952 book *Black Skin, White Masks*. As a result, he championed the importance of understanding a people's historical context in order to provide them with ethical and efficacious services. In his 1961 work, *The Wretched of the Earth*, Fanon extrapolates that decolonization is an inherently violent process in that the colonized are justified to fight oppression with violence absent reverence to general principles of humanity because the colonizers don't see them as human. Regarding the natural process of decolonization, he writes that violence "is a cleansing force. It frees the native from his inferiority complex and from his despair and inaction; it makes him fearless and restores his self-respect" (Oliver, 2004, p. 59). Fanon would become a voice of African liberation, initially within the context of French colonialism in Algeria and then in general. Fanon's philosophy would serve as one of several grounding principles for the American Black Power and Liberation Movements which would move the model of justice from one of civil disobedience to Black liberation and political autonomy (Jooste, 2009; Oliver, 2004).

St Benedict the Moor was born in Sicily in 1526. His parents were brought to the Italian island as enslaved people, but his freedom was secured prior to his birth as a result of his parents "loyal service". Early on he dedicated his life to the service and relief of those less fortunate. He would eventually give away all his possessions and join a religious order where he grew a reputation for his theological understanding and knowledge of the scripture. He was often sought after for counsel, much like Dr. Martin Luther King Jr. who was also revered for his service, dedication to the less fortunate along with his deep theological knowledge base. Born over 400 years apart in separate parts of the world, these men would both die on April 4th leaving a legacy of justice and equity for all people.

Shaka Zulu, born in 1787, was one of the most significant Black rulers and warriors in the history of the world. Although not immediately seen as a noteworthy or revered leader, he would rise in popularity and influence after the death of his mentor, Dingiswayo. Shaka would move south and establish a new capitol where military might and expertise would generate increase in the kingdom's cultural reach and capacity to rule. Malcolm X was born in 1925 and was one of the America's most significant Black civil rights warriors. He fought vehemently for the rights of Black people specifically. He too was initially unpopular but gained notoriety as he grew and developed. He would establish temples of worship in many different US cities where his powerful warrior like oratory skills were revered. Both Malcolm and Shaka would be assassinated by men who they considered brothers.

Aimé Césaire was a French poet and politician born in the French colony of Martinique in 1913. His leadership led to the French Négritude Movement in literature and politics. Along with men like Léopold Senghor and Léon Dama, Césaire renounced European colonialism and fought for the philosophies of Pan-Africanism. The Négritude Movement would birth several diasporic philosophies including the American Black is Beautiful movement that worked to counter Eurocentric paradigms of beauty which consistently rendered images of Blackness as not simply unattractive, but ugly. In 1935, Césaire, a student at Paris' elite and highly selective École normale supérieure, created a literary review called L'Ètudiante Noir (The Black Student) for which Senghor and Dama were contributors (Rabaka, 2015).

There are endless permutations of Black male strength that one could pronounce. The cross-continental associations and connections between them have been deliberately and purposefully broken. Elijah McCoy and Garrett Morgan mechanized innovation, while Medgar Evers and Marcus Garvey inspired people to move, literally and figuratively. Talib Kweli, Wiley and Samy Deluxe spoke the language of a generation that many attempted to silence, while Ira Aldridge and Laurence Fishburne graced the stage with Shakespearean prose demonstrating an expertise that shocked many. Olaudah Equiano and Frederick Douglass catalyzed their respective abolitionist's movements, while Dr. Anderson Ruffin Abbott and Dr. James McCune Smith were bold enough to become medical practitioners when no one said they could. Each of these men held allegiances to national identities that differed from one another, yet they share in their Africanness a common bond concealed to maintain both distance and detachment from one another. One doesn't naturally see the connections between the Bantu Migration across Africa and the Great Migration across America, or the energy from the Harlem Renaissance traveling the ocean to inspire the Negritude movement in France, which volleyed back to spark the Black Power Movement. The necessary fortitude of a people is born from the synergy of connectedness that provides evidence of efficacy and agency while strengthening the soul.

ORIGINS OF MAN AND ITS FAMILIES

This vast continent is not only the definitive seat of all civilizations, it also houses in its land great wealth, wealth that outsiders would eventually go to great lengths to acquire. Gold, ivory, diamonds, people, medicine and science were but a few of the goods rumored to flank the continent in ancient times. Magnificent stories of gold, jewels, ivory and people with exotic Black skin saturated the known world of the time. These stories created a magnetic force for nations seeking wealth, power and influence during medieval times, a magnetism that would eventually operationalize itself as one of the world's greatest atrocities.

The continent of Africa has seen the rise and fall of many kingdoms throughout its long and rich history. Due to the climatic diversity of the continent, Africans had been trading among one another for millennia. Each group played a very specific role; desert nomads brought salt, meats and fish from the Niger river. The forest-dwellers contributed furs and meat. Hunter gatherers bought the expertise of herding and foraging to pastoral communities. This collaboration, their shared knowledge and the domestication of important livestock and crops led to the start of several relatively static communities.

The surprisingly well-documented migration of and interactions among African people across the continent began on some large scale millennia ago. In order to do appropriate justice to this text and maintain the integrity of its scope, this exploration begins with a cursory look at life and continental migration in the years Before Common Era (BCE) to contextualize the histories of the Common Era (CE) cultures across the continent. Ten thousand years ago, over what we know today as the Sahara Desert, monsoon rains fell creating a lush habitable land mass for people, vegetation and wild life to thrive. This lasted for millennia until around 3500 BCE when the overused land was met with less rain fall and devolved back into the pre-monsoon arid Sahara of today. The people of various cultural and linguistic traditions who lived in this region were forced to migrate for survival. Some moved closer to the banks of the Nile while others moved in different directions. Part of this group is responsible for the start of the well-studied Egyptian pharaonic era around 3100 BCE (Newman, 1995).

Bodies of research reference the existence of three regional genetic populations from which virtually all Africans descend: The, Capoid, Congoid and Caucasoid. Evidence—primarily from cranial morphology—demonstrates that these proto-populations had been formed by the end of Africa's Late Stone Age. The Capoid and the Congoid races, each inclusive of several "sub-races", have historically been aggregated into one Negroid race in anthropological research. Each of these groups and their sub-races are explored further throughout the course of this chapter. Their descendants were subsequently categorized into cultural groups using multi-disciplinary data and evidence from three major domains (McEvedy, 1995; Meredith, 2014; Newman, 1995).

- Common characteristics found across their languages.
- The geographic region where their remains were discovered.
- Lifestyle evidence including but not limited to nomadic patterns, crop records, tools utilized and geographically related animal fossils.

Each of these domains has been explored within and across a multitude of scientific spheres. As a result, the origins of many contemporary African nations, tribes and cultures can be traced along very specific linguistic, geographic and behavioral patterns.

Paleolinguists, archaeo-anthropologist and ethno-archaeologists juxtapose the historical records of language and communication with that of fossils and artifacts to support hypotheses about the cultural connectivity among ancient groups of people. Historical linguistics and archaeology are used together to reconstruct proto-language geneses and pre-historic migratory patterns. Together, these confirmations help to develop evidence-based ethno-graphic connections. Proto-languages or parent languages diverged into new dialects and languages based on a variety of factors across time (Holden, 2002; Perreault & Mathew, 2012).

Lexicostatistics is one of several tools used by linguists to analyze percentages of phonemes and words in a language that share a common etymology to understand when and potentially where that particular language or dialect diverged from the proto-language. This process was commonly employed to classify the myriad of ancient African populations into common speech communities and ethno-linguistic cultural groups. All languages have a point of origin, and they tend to evolve in a manner that is both predictable and observable. All the languages—over 1000—spoken on the African continent have origins traced to four ethno-linguistic phyla: Khoisan, Niger–Congo, Nilo-Saharan and Afro-Asiatic. Each phylum is further divided into families that share commonalities in their core vocabularies and grammar. Each family includes an array of languages and dialects (Holden, 2002; Perreault & Mathew, 2012).

Pre-colonial communities across Africa, including merchants, nobles, farmers, traders and warriors, all originate from one of these ethno-linguistic families. When a group of people share the ability to communicate with one another, the foundation for community—in both the tangible and esoteric sense—is built. Through the addition of the prefix ethno—to the term ethno-linguistic family—researchers implicate a set of shared beliefs, worldviews, cultural traditions and social value systems that synergize with a shared language and ability to communicate with one another. As a result of this synergy, ethnically unified groups often referred to as tribes are created. While there are several ways to explore the history of the continent's people and its empires, following the events experienced by some of the people in each of the ethno-linguistic phyla and their interactions with one another across time provides a non-chronological yet effective perspective into the pre-colonial state of the African continent.

It has become common place to isolate the heritages of contemporary Black men and women across the diaspora as having descended solely from the Western regions of the continent. Although countries like current day Senegal, Cote d'Ivoire and Ghana represent some of the primary trading posts and kidnapping grounds for enslavers and colonizers, the contemporary African diaspora has very diverse roots, as did the stolen souls of their ancestors. Their trauma-ridden transatlantic journey may have commenced across a reportedly constricted swath of the continent's geography, but their origins are not nearly as singular as we have been instructed to believe.

Khoisan Family

The Khoisan phylum is the smallest ethno-linguistic phyla and includes the language families of Khoikhoi and San people. Based on nuclear genetic testing, the Khoisan ethno-linguistic groups represent the most ancient genetic divergence from the original African phylogenetic root across both patrilineal (Y Chromosome) and matrilineal (mitochondrial DNA) lines (Pickrell & Reich, 2014). The Khoisan people, pejoratively known in historical literature as the Hottentots, represent the collective ethno-cultural identity of both the Khoikhoi and San people who migrated south prior to the Bantu Expansion. The Khoisan people are known for the notable "click" sound that permeates most phonemic aspects of their language. Khoisan is a contemporary anthropological convention which aggregates these descendants of the earliest anatomically modern humans who migrated to the southern portion of Africa millennia ago (Zimmer, 2016).

The San people are the earliest known hunter-gatherer communities on the continent of Africa. Records of their existence in Southern Africa demonstrate at least 20,000 years of inhabitation in the region. They were formerly known as Bushmen by the Europeans, a descriptor currently considered deprecating and no longer in use. Khoikhoi people originated in modern-day Botswana and migrated south as they mastered the pastoral lifestyle. The Khoisan people of southern Africa host the largest genetic diversity in a world where contemporary humans share over 99% of the same genome. In one study, Southern Africans represented over 2 million DNA variables per individual, the largest ever (American Association for the Advancement of Sciences, 2012).

NIGER–CONGO FAMILY

The Niger–Congo ethno-linguistic phyla include over 1300 languages and dialects in families that include: Bantu, Adamawa, Mande, Atlantic, Kwa and Voltaic. The specific languages in these families include Ewe, Yoruba, Somali, Dogon, Xhosi, Mossi and Soninke (Newman, 1995). It is identified as Africa's largest language phyla, and as of 2015, data confirmed that the 700 million people of the Niger–Congo ethno-linguistic phyla also cover an expansive geographic region across the continent. Members of this group occupied territories from the Senegal River in northern Senegal to the southeast in modern-day Cameroon (Zimmer, 2016).

Ghana was one of West Africa's first kingdoms, reigning from the sixth to the thirteenth century and playing a critical role in the entire history of western Africa. Situated perfectly—geographically and socially—Ghana developed great wealth and power as a major player in the trade of salt, gold, people and textiles. The trans-Saharan trade route connected merchants and their markets across the Sahara from the Mediterranean to the Niger River delta. The Ghanaian people were of Soninke origin and referred to their kingdom as Wagadu; the name Ghana was given by the Arabs of the time. One of the kingdoms most famous cities and its likely capital was Koumbi. Ghanaian kingdoms grew from the Neolithic Dhar Tichitt communities in Southern Mauretania inhabited by pastoralist as early as 4000 BCE during the slow evolution from hunter-gatherer communities in the region. Climatic changes impacted these agro-pastoral communities leaving the land barren except for oases scattered here and there. These areas were re-settled by iron using communities during the first half century AD and share a striking resemblance to Koumbi Saleh (McIntosh, 2008; Meyerowitz, 1952; Munson, 1980).

Much of the trade happening in and around the kingdom of Ghana was related to the North African Berber (Afro-Asiatic ethno-linguistic family) caravans traveling across the Sahara from the Maghreb. In addition to a substantial supply of gold, the Ghanaian kings mastered the art of trade and built a successful system that incorporated routes from the Mediterranean, the Atlantic, the Maghreb, Egypt, Arabia, Spain and even India. They created systems of measurement, patterns of trade and even charged a tax on all imports and exports. The Ghanaian militia was large, well trained and expertly developed. They created safe trade routes and provided private security—at a cost—when requested during trading. All these factors combined catalyzed the kingdom's ascension to great wealth and power. Due to the successful Trans-Saharan systems of trade, Ghana was not only wealthy, it served as a point of convergence for ideas, technology, culture and the foundations of a citizenry focused on efforts beyond mere survival. This success would last for centuries until jealous and/or opportunistic nations successfully attacked the region for its seemingly limitless supply of gold and its monopoly on trade (McIntosh, 2008; Meyerowitz, 1952; Munson, 1980).

In 1076, its capital would be destroyed by the Almoravids, a group of Muslim Berbers and Arabs from Northern Africa. The extent to which the Almoravids devastated the kingdom is unclear. Some indicate that evidence of such a sudden change attributable to Almoravid military advances during this era is inexistent. Others cite the source(s) of the evidence on which we base Ghana's history—primarily of Arab narrative and account—as potentially slanted toward an exaggeration of success for the Muslim Almoravids. Others state that the 1076 event was minor and that Ghana would reclaim prominence, pushing the Berbers out for almost 200 more years. According to almost all accounts, however, by the end of the first quarter of the thirteenth century, many of the original citizens had fled, and just a few short years later, Sundiata, ruler of the kingdom of Mali, destroyed what remained of Ghana and named himself ruler (McIntosh, 2008).

The Niger–Congo phyla also included the Benue Kwa people, whose direct descendants consist of the Bantu, the Yoruba, the Igbo and the Akan. The Bantu people currently make up over half of the Niger–Congo speaking people in Africa. Although European colonists encountered the Bantu people while in Southern Africa, their origins were thousands of miles north. Mapping their migration (east and south), often referred to as the Bantu Expansion, opens a provocative window into the ancient history of Africa, its people and their varied interactions and engagements. As climates changed, livestock were domesticated and metal working became a skill set, many aspects of life began to change. Trade commenced across the regions of the continent, and areas became increasingly populated. The African people migrated all across the continent and went on to populate the world as we know it today. Iron work was pervasive in east Africa, speeding the migration of the Bantu people to the southern parts of the continent throughout 1000 BCE. The Bantu people migrated both east and south, trading with and creating families among the native tribes they encountered on their treks (Holden, 2002).

According to paleoanthropologists, native hunter-gatherer and pastoral populations thrived across the continent prior to the Bantu Expansion. The Bantu groups who traveled south would meet and build community with the San and Khoikhoi. Those who traveled east encountered the ancient BaTwa hunter-gatherers of central Africa, commonly known as the Pygmies. As direct descendants of the Middle Stone Age (MSA) hunter-gatherers, the BaTwa represent the second most ancient genetic divergence from the original African phylogenetic root. The MSA hunter-gatherers were in fact anatomically modern human beings unlike the Neanderthals that inhabited Europe during their Middle Paleolithic Era (MPE). Although these time periods (MSA and MPE) are often referenced interchangeably in that they cover the exact same chronological time period, the nuanced distinction honors the literal different stages of human development and cognition occurring on each continent during these time periods (Holden, 2002).

AFRO-ASIATIC FAMILY

The Afro-asiatic ethno-linguistic group includes the Berbers, the Chadic, the Semitic, the Egyptian and the (K)Cushitic people. The primary languages spoken among this group include Somali, Arabic, Hebrew, Oromo and Hausa (Newman, 1995). It is noted that this group of Africans were in communities juxtaposed to the Nilo-Saharans to the south. King Alara is often credited with initiating the reunification of Egypt and placing the capital at Napata. Archeological evidence has not fully supported his role as a pharaoh but recognized his contribution to the origins of the 25th Dynasty. Upon his death, his brother, Kashta, became the king of Upper and Lower Egypt after forming a close alliance with Thebes. He named his daughter, Amenirdis I, to one of the most prominent political roles in the kingdom. Serving as their god's Divine Adoretress of Amun (high priestess), they worshipped her role and subsequently cemented the religious traditions with the political body (Barrat, 2014; Newman, 1995).

Under the leadership of King Piye—Kashta's son—the 25th Dynasty officially began. He was a strategic and decisive military man conquering Upper, Middle and Lower Egypt. Piye was a devout worshipper of Amun as were most other Kushites of the time. In times of battle, he would offer sacrifices to Amun and regularly require his soldiers to engage in ritualistic cleansings prior to battle. Documented festivals of Ancient Egypt worshipping deities and Gods of the Kushite people considered along with the fossil and archaeological record prove the prominence of this dynasty as they proceeded north to the Lower Nile Valley to take over all of Egypt. Piye and his troops successfully took the Egyptian cities of Hermopolis and Memphis—major cultural centers of ancient times—forcing the submission of the Nile Delta kings. A distinction is made here for the 25th dynasty, not because they are uniquely more African than the pharaohs preceding or following them, but because they have been consistently identified as foreign pharaohs when they actually share a common ethno-linguistic phylum with other celebrated pharaohs (American Association for the Advancement of Science, 2012; Harkless, 2006; Newman, 1995).

King Piye was the ruler of Upper Egypt, to the south, and was able to take advantage of the intradynastic fighting that was occurring in Lower Egypt (in the north) where the Nile spreads the arms of its delta into the Mediterranean Sea. Shabaka, his brother, would rule after Piye passed away in Nubia. Not only did he rule the nation, he successfully merged the cultures and was known as the ruler of both Kush and Egypt. He built temples, pyramids and the Treasury of Shabaka. He is even credited for the restoration of ancient Egyptian historic symbols in Thebes and Carnac and the Shabaka stone (also known as the Memphite Theology) which discusses and documents the history of Ancient Egypt. Although he effectively resisted the first assault of the Assyrians, it would be Shebitku who actually battled them for the first time as they sieged westward toward Egypt. Tantamani, nephew of Taharqa, was the last pharaoh of the 25th dynasty. The Nubian kings and Kushite culture would continue in the Sudan and Upper Egypt for over 10,000 years through 370 CE. Assyrian rule would be followed by the Persians and then two Hellenistic dynasties with Alexander the Great and then the Ptolemaic Dynasty after that. The Kushites merged Egyptian ethos with theirs, creating a unique culture that would thrive for centuries. They unified the country of Egypt and minimized attacks from the Berbers of Libya who had long divided the area. The Kushites would thrive in Upper Egypt for many generations trading with the various ruling groups until they were finally weakened by the Romans under the rule of Emperor Augustus (American Association for the Advancement of Science, 2012; Harkless, 2006; Newman, 1995; United Nations Educational, Scientific and Cultural Organization [UNESCO], 1990).

The Imazighen, better known as the Berbers—from the Latin *barbarous* meaning barbarian—of Northern Africa, evolved from early ethnolinguistic Afro-Asiatic groups around 5000 BCE. Engagements of trade, conquest and counter-conquest with the Romans, the Arabs, the Egyptians and the Europeans throughout the years would play a significant role in the cultural and economic development of the Berber populations across northern Africa. Meshwesh and Ribu are two of the most noteworthy groups of Berbers. The North African Berbers were pushed from their region and enslaved by the Phoenicians fleeing Alexander the Great's annexation of Tyre, one of Phoenicia's most powerful states. In 332 BCE, tens of thousands of Tyrians were massacred and/or enslaved by Alexander and his militia; others were able to use their wealth to escape his fatal wrath. Many of these men and women fled to Carthage, a Phoenician state across the Mediterranean in North Africa established by Queen Dido in 814 BCE after she was exiled from Tyre (Newman, 1995; Vernus & Yoyotte, 2003).

At the establishment of Carthage, the Berbers had already mastered agricultural techniques that often lead nomadic communities to more sedentary and pastoral ones. Two prominent Berber regions neighboring

Carthage were Numidia and Mauretania. For many years, the Berbers and the Phoenicians in Carthage got along well in their trading and neighborly engagement. There was even a notable population of Berbers in Carthage by this time, some served in the Phoenician military, but most were relegated to a lower hierarchical existence beneath the Phoenicians. Masinissa, a western Numidian Berber raised in Carthage, was the son of Numidian tribal chief Gala. He would become one of the region's most notable rulers. As a young soldier, he led Carthage into victory against Syphax and the Masaesyli of eastern Numidia who were allies with Rome. He would make considerable contributions to Carthaginian victories in 211 BCE by leading a group of Numidian soldiers against the Roman advances in nearby Spain. His leadership and battle acumen were so significant that he was placed in command of the entire Carthaginian cavalry in Spain (American Association for the Advancement of Sciences, 2012; Vernus & Yoyotte, 2003).

The Battle of Ilipa (206 BCE), where Scipio Africanus' crafty warmanship overwhelmed Masinissa and the Phoenicians, effectively shifted the course of the region's history. He effectively pushed Carthage their influence and their forces out of the Iberian Peninsula. This was a critical moment for Masinissa. He was able to see the writing on the wall so to speak and shifted his allegiance. After years and dedication to Carthage, Masinissa would go on to lead the Massylii Numidia—one of the most powerful Berber tribes—after defecting to Rome in the third century BCE (Hoyos, 2017; Vernus & Yoyotte, 2003).

During the Punic Wars between the Romans and the Carthaginians, the Massylii kingdom would partner with the Romans to defeat Carthage. In 202 BCE, Masinissa led thousands of Roman and Numidian soldiers in the Battle of Zama. Their successful defeat of Carthage ended the 2nd Punic war and solidified Masinissa's status as a remarkable, battle-tested military expert. For his efforts, the western region of Numidia was annexed to him, uniting both the Massylii and Masaesyli into one Numidia under Roman jurisdiction. Masinissa would continue to expand his power as cities grew, technology advanced and sedentary agriculture became more prevalent. The capital city of Cirta thrived as it innovated ways of living, advanced systems of trade and facilitated complex international relationships. Masinissa's empire grew as he and his sons acquired large estates across Northern Africa. During this time, his intentions also became clearer and increasingly threatening. The goal of uniting all of Northern Africa under his rule was evident, and the Roman

Empire—likely waiting for the aging king to die—was surely strategizing to minimize any uprisings from the Numidians in the land that remained a vassal of the Roman Empire (American Association for the Advancement of Sciences, 2012; Barrat, 2014; Vernus & Yoyotte, 2003; UNESCO, 1990).

In the middle of the second century BCE, Rome encouraged Numidia to provoke Carthage into war, and Numidian soldiers were deployed to Carthage. They burned down towns, attacked villages and utterly terrorized the Carthaginians. Under any other circumstances, the clear and most present response would be to retaliate; this was unfortunately not so cut and dry. A portion of the peace treaty between Carthage and Rome barred them from waging war against any nation—even if provoked—without permission from Rome. When the Phoenicians reciprocated the Numidian attack, they effectively broke the treaty, placing them in direct violation of their agreement. Roman soldiers descended upon Northern Africa, and Carthage was the destination. Masinissa, hoping to annex Carthage for Numidia, was dismayed by the 149 BCE arrival of the Roman army but died the following year at almost 90 years old (Hoyos, 2017).

After King Masinissa, King Jugurtha ascended the throne and would eventually be captured and killed by the Romans in the first major conflict between Numidia and Rome. Chieftain Juba II united the Berbers of Numidia with the neighboring Berbers of Mauretania against Caesar during the Great Roman Civil War. Although they were not victorious, the Berber identity would remain functional and distinctive even after generations under Roman rule. In fact, the Berbers of Mauretania—often called the Mauri—are the direct ancestors of the North African Moors who would occupy the Iberian Peninsula, Sicily and the Maghreb throughout the Middle Ages. In 1052, Arab warriors and nomads from the Banu Hilal and Banu Sulaym tribes migrated west from Egypt to conquer the Berber people whose culture would be eventually absorbed during what became known as the Hilalian invasion. Arab language, culture and religion would spread across northern Africa, changing it forever (Etheredge, 2010).

Traveling through Europe, it is easy to see the ancient qualities of the architecture and infrastructure that abound. Walking through the streets of Malaga, one of the oldest cities in the world, provides an amazing context. Standing on the coast of Europe's most southern major city, one can almost feel the history that occurred along those shores. Fellowshipping with the people of the small neighboring towns that make up the province like Fuengirola, Mijas and Marbella creates a literal proxy to the ancestral spirits of the Castilians, Arabs and Africans who once were a part of this Andalusian community on the Iberian Peninsula. Black soldiers of the time who specifically identified as Moors were vigorously conscripted by Rome and served in other European militias including but not limited to Britain, France and Switzerland. St. Maurice, patron saint of medieval Europe, is often commemorated throughout German churches as an African Roman soldier. He was one of many Black soldiers with allegiance to the Roman Empire. The Moorish advances in disciplines like mathematics, astronomy, hydraulic engineering, art and agriculture helped to move Europe out of the Dark Ages and into the Renaissance. In the tenth century, Cordoba, the capital of Moorish Spain at the time, was one of the most influential cities in the world. Its population was approximately a half million people. They had street lighting, hospitals, mosques and libraries. In addition to those innovations, they introduced new crops to the region and developed grain storage practices. During this time, London and Paris had not yet seen such advances as those of the Roman Empire had been allowed to disappear for the most part. Many believe that the growth and development of European intellectualism was born after they visited libraries and learning centers in Moor-controlled Spain and returned home to emulate the structures (Atlanta Black Star, 2013; EU Travel Magazine, 2017; Lamb, 2013).

NILO-SAHARAN FAMILY

Nilo-Saharan ethno-linguistic phylum includes Sudanic, Saharan and Songhai families. The people of this ethno-linguistic group live in almost 20 different nations in the northern part of the continent from Algeria in the west to Tanzania in the east covering the greater Nile basin and the central portions of the Sahara. The major languages of this linguistic family include Nubian, Songhai, Nandi, Luo and Nuer. The 50–60 million people speaking languages represented in this group have histories that have impacted global affairs of religion, finance and politics. Nubia was one of Africa's busiest international meeting points, a place where Greeks, Romans, Arabs, Assyrians and other Africans would intermingle through trade and commerce. The Songhai Empire and its capital at Timbuktu represent one of western Africa's most prominent systems of rulers and intellects. The Dholuo-speaking people of Kenya and Tanzania along with the Nuer-speaking people of Ethiopia and the Sudan are all parts of Africa's lesser known pre-colonial puzzles (Graham, 1987; Newman, 1995).

In the Ethiopian village of Yeha stands the Temple of the Moon, a pre-Christian temple where parishioners worshipped during the same time in history when the Old Testament prophets were said to have been documenting the occurrences of the time. Archaeologists believe it is the oldest building in Ethiopia dating back to about 700 BC, older than the Parthenon, the Coliseum and the Erechtheion. The Kebra Nagast is one of the world's most under-revered historical religious books in the world. According to some, it is the Christian Bible imbued with Ethiopian history detailing the Solomonic Dynasty. It includes the stories of Queen Makeda of Ethiopia—the Queen of Sheba—meeting King Solomon and bearing their child, Melenik. It discusses his return to Ethiopia with the Ark of the Covenant before the Babylonian Empire invaded Jerusalem and conquered Israel. According to Christian tradition, the Ark of the Covenant is thought to hold the stone tablets of the Ten Commandments and is rumored to be held at St. Mary of Zion cathedral in the Ethiopian city of Aksum (Britannica, Solomonid, 2018b; Newman, 1995; Raffaele, 2007).

Egypt (Kemet), after over a millennium of successful rule and dominance, was weakened by the Axum people of Ethiopia, who had come to power after the debilitated Kushite Kingdom began its declined. Ezana, the first Ethiopian Christian king of Axum, defeated the Kushites in the fourth century and ruled the Axum kingdom, made up of present-day Ethiopia, Yemen, Somalia, Djibouti, Eritrea and the Sudan. The Ezana Stone monument, a multi-lingual proclamation demonstrating the king's strength and commemorating the conquering of nations in the name of Christianity, exists today in Ethiopia's city of Axum. One of the languages on the stone is an archaic language from Saba, a region in Yemen where the Queen of Sheba is said to have been from (Graham, 1987; Newman, 1995; Raffaele, 2007).

Although there were several kings and rulers of Ethiopia that followed Ezana, Kaleb of Axum is one of the most noteworthy and well documented. In the early sixth century, Kaleb and his troops took southern Arabia defeating the Jewish Dhu Nuwas of Himyarite (current day Yemen) who had been persecuting Christians throughout the region, even threatening to secede from the rest of the region. During the reign of Kaleb, the Axumites controlled traffic throughout the Red Sea, created monopoly-like systems of trade with countries in the Far East and developed one of the mightiest military powers in the region. Known for protecting Christians from persecution and conquering overseas land, Kaleb became the first Ethiopian canonized by the Greek and Roman Catholic Churches. He is known as St. Elesbaan in the Roman Martyrology, a list of Saints identified by the Roman Church. These Black Axum kings created and operated sophisticated systems of international trade with the Romans, the Egyptians and the Arabs. They used their land's wealth of natural resources (wheat, barley, gold, emeralds, etc.) strategically to sustain a system that gave them notoriety across the known and developed land (Graham, 1987; Newman, 1995).

The Zagwe Dynasty would follow the Axumites as the next set of generational rulers and cultural influencers of the land. Ethiopia has not been sufficiently excavated and studied, resulting in an archaeological gap in the historical record. Accounts of Queen Judith—sometimes known as the Queen of the Ethiopian Jews—ruling the land and destroying the Axum kingdom's capital in the late ninth century seem to be consistently supported across multiple accounts prior to the ascendance of the Zagwe Dynasty. Researchers suggest that the continuity and refinement of Axum traditions and architecture within Zagwe rule is indicative of either: the brevity with which any group reigned in between the two or the deliberate elimination from collective memory of the great terror wielded by those intermediate rulers. Whatever combination turns out to be true, it is well-documented that the Zagwe Dynasty left a marked impression on the entire region and known world of the time (Negash, 2008).

Yemrehanna Krestos, Zagwe ruler of the late twelfth century, was the first to define land borders according to the Apostolic Canons. He built his palace and church inside the mouth of a large cave within the Ethiopian Highlands where a natural lake ran through it. A very rich land, more crop species are found in the Ethiopian Highlands than other area on the continent. Krestos' brother, King Lalibela, would ascend to the throne after him, moving the capitol to Roha where he built a multitude of churches and ornate housing for the priestly class likely supported by peasants and pilgrims. It is storied that King Gebre Mesqel Lalibela's birth was christened by God through the swarming of bees around his new born body. As an adult, the story continues that he had a dream where God told him to rebuild Jerusalem in Ethiopia and the 11 churches of Lalibela were born. Models of carving expertise using progressive technology of the time, each church required the excavation of tons of stone without the use of modern mechanization. With expert precision, they were artistically carved downward into the bedrock near to the water table, requiring a great deal of both architectural and engineering proficiency. Although the construction and design of the churches hold influences from international trade partners, religious comrades and local political allies, they remain as unique architectural fetes of the modern world. Roha would be renamed Lalibela posthumously after its ruler of 40 years and remains today one of Ethiopia's most contemporarily pilgrimaged locations where people collect the soil and sand as it is said to have healing qualities (Graham, 1987; MacEachern, 2000; McEvedy, 1995; Negash, 2008).

During the last half of the thirteenth century, Yekuno Amiak would defeat the last Zagwe king to re-establish the Solomonic rule of Ethiopia. Amiak, an Amhara prince, would even claim specific ancestral lineage to the last Solomonic Axum king to reign prior to the Zagwe Dynasty, Dil Na'od. Although the Solomonic aristocracy ruled from decentralized locations to maintain protection of their vast borders, they secured strong trading relationships with both Egypt and Jerusalem. Rulers would have caravans of tens of thousands of people following them from place to place across seasons, impacting urbanism and the development of sustainable cities in the region (Graham, 1987; Negash, 2008).

In Conclusion

The historical record is undeniable, and this collective body of evidence is incontestable. Even with all these facts, the propensity to negate and revise the histories of Black men across the diaspora continues to grow endemically. Even in the context of the often revered ancient Roman societies, Black Africans played significant roles, but their stories were often vilified. Black African Roman emperors like Septimius Severus born in present-day Libya are rarely spoken of. He was raised in Northern Africa and educated in Rome. He was a lawyer, a Roman Senator and a governor before ruling the Roman Empire from 193 to 211 CE. He was a deliberate and decisive ruler who is ignored throughout much of Roman history. The story of his son, Caracalla, is one of even greater relevance to this body of research. Caracalla would rule jointly with his father for some time and then his brother after that. He would become the sole Roman Emperor following their deaths.

Roman Emperors like Constantine, Pius and Vespasian are well known, studied and celebrated, yet most will never learn about this noble father–son dyad of African descent who ruled Rome across two generations. Research shows a great deal of ambiguity in perceptions of Caracalla, but what is most clear are the efforts across disciplines that characterize him as a vicious tyrant with a mental health disorder. Caracalla would work to further strengthen the empire as did his father before him, yet he would be painted as a murderous deviant. When one searches for images of Caracalla, they are more often than not confronted with a bust of a man with tightly coiled hair and the most unapproachable scowl one has ever seen (Syvänne, 2017).

This congruence across history to develop, sustain and strengthen a system where stories of Black male forte, intellect, compassion and resilience are omitted or revised is striking. Pre-dating Biblical antiquity through contemporary modernity, the history of African noble ancestry has been clouded and cloaked from our origin stories. This serves as a significant barrier to the foundations of a cultural group's wellness. All are responsible for ensuring that learners from different backgrounds fight against supremacy's compelling forces at work to minimize pre-enslavement and pre-colonial value. Was Caracalla a bad man? The ambiguities in the research seem to think so and cast him as such. There are, however, an array of men across historical contexts with both prosocial and anti-social characteristics, and a close look demonstrates that their legacies are often bifurcated along lines drawn upon phenotypic characteristics, skin color in this instance. Deliberately denying the opportunity to ensure that Black children are familiar with their entire historical context and relevance is a silent endorsement aimed at maintaining their oppression across generations.

References

American Association for the Advancement of Science. (2012). *Khoe-San Peoples Are Unique, Special-Largest Genomic Study Finds.* University of the Witwatersrand. Retrieved April 29, 2018, from https://www.eurekalert.org/pub_releases/2012-09/uotw-kpa091412.php

Atlanta Black Star. (2013). *When Black Men Ruled the World: 8 Things The Moors Brought to Europe.*

Barrat, J. (2014). *Rise of the Black Pharaohs.* Documentary. PBS 55min.

Bosshard, P. (2011). *New Chinese Dam Project Fuels Ethnic Conflict in Sudan.* International Rivers. Retrieved from https://www.internationalrivers.org/blogs/227/new-chinese-dam-project-fuels-ethnic-conflict-in-sudan

Bower, B. (2017). Oldest Known *Homo Sapien* Fossils Come from Northern Africa, Studies Claim. *Magazine of the Society for Science and the Public.*

Cavalli-Sforza, L. L., Menozzi, P., & Piazza, A. (1994). *The History and Geography of Human Genes.* Princeton, NJ: Princeton University Press.

Encyclopedia Britannica. (2018a). *Olduvai Gorge.* Retrieved from https://www.britannica.com/place/Olduvai-Gorge

Encyclopedia Britannica. (2018b). *Solomonid Dynasty.* Retrieved from https://www.britannica.com/topic/Solomonid-dynasty

Enough. (2016). *Nubians Protest Nile River Dams.* Retrieved from https://enoughproject.org/blog/nubians-protest-nile-river-dams

Etheredge, L. (Ed.). (2010). *The Islamic World: Islamic History.* New York: Britannica Educational Publishing.

EU Travel Magazine. (2017). *In the Footsteps of the Moors: Cordoba.* Retrieved from http://www.e-travelmag.com/spain/in-the-footsteps-of-the-moors-cordoba/

Gibbons, A. (2016, February 17). *Humans Mated with Neanderthals Much Earlier and More Frequently Than Thought.* Retrieved July 30, 2018, from http://www.sciencemag.org/news/2016/02/humans-mated-neandertals-much-earlier-and-more-frequently-thought

Graham, C. (1987). *African Civilizations: Precolonial Cities and States in Tropical Africa: An Archaeological Perspective.* New York: Cambridge University Press.

Harkless, N. (2006). *Nubian Pharaohs and Meroitic Kings: The Kingdom of Kush.* Bloomington, IN: Authorhouse.

Hawkins, J., Elliott, M., Schmid, P., Churchill, S. E., Ruiter, D. J., Roberts, E. M., et al. (2017). New Fossil Remains of Homo Naledi from the Lesedi Chamber, South Africa. *Genomics and Evolutionary Biology.* Retrieved from https://elifesciences.org/articles/24232 on 4/29/18

Holden, C. J. (2002). Bantu Language Trees Reflect the Spread of Farming Across Sub-Saharan Africa: A Maximum-Parsimony Analysis. *Proceedings of the Royal Society of London. Series B: Biological Sciences, 269*(1493), 793–799.

Hoyos, B. D. (2017). *Mastering the West: Rome and Carthage at War.* New York: Oxford University Press.

Hublin, J. J. (2017). New Fossils from Jebel Irhoud, Morocco and the Pan-African Origin of Homo sapiens. *Nature, 546,* 289–292.

Jooste, R. J. (2009). *Fanon, Frantz (1925–1961). The International Encyclopedia of Revolution and Protest.*

Kuhlwilm, M., & Gronau, I. (2016). Ancient Gene Flow from Early Modern Humans into Eastern Neanderthals. *Nature, 530,* 429–433.

Lamb, J. (2013). *Black.* Bloomington, IN: Authorhouse.

Lemieux, P. (2018). *The Silver Lining.* Library of Economics & Liberty. Retrieved from https://www.econlib.org/the-silver-lining-of-negationism/

MacEachern, S. (2000). Genes, Tribes and African History. *Current Anthropology, 41*(3), 357–384.

Martin, M. (2018). Slave Bible from the 1800s Omitted Key Passages That Could Incite Rebellion. *NPR.* Retrieved from https://www.npr.org/2018/12/09/674995075/slave-bible-from-the-1800s-omitted-key-passages-that-could-incite-rebellion

McEvedy, C. (1995). *The Penguin Atlas of African History.* London: Penguin.

McIntosh, S. (2008). Reconceptualizing Early Ghana. *Canadian Journal of African Studies/Revue Canadienne Des Études Africaines, 42*(2/3), 347–373. Retrieved from http://www.jstor.org/stable/40380172

Meredith, M. (2014). *The Fortunes of Africa: A 5000-Year History of Wealth, Greed and Endeavor.* New York: Public Affairs.

Meyerowitz, E. L. R. (1952). A Note on the Origins of Ghana. *African Affairs, 51*(205), 319–323. Retrieved from http://www.jstor.org/stable/718785

Munson, J. P. (1980). Archaeology and Prehistoric Origins of the Ghana Empire. *Journal of African History, 21*(4), 457–466.

Negash, T. (2008). *The Zagwe Period Re-Interpreted: Post-Aksumite Ethiopian Urban Culture.* Retrieved from https://www.arkeologi.uu.se/digitalAssets/36/c_36108-l_3-k_negashall.pdf

Newman, J. L. (1995). *The Peopling of Africa: A Geographic Interpretation.* New Haven, CT: Yale University Press.

Oliver, K. (2004). *The Colonization of Psychic Space: A Psychoanalytic Social Theory of Oppression.* Minneapolis, MN: University of Minnesota Press.

Oppenheimer, S. (2012). Out-of-Africa, the Peopling of Continents and Islands: Tracing Uniparental Genes Trees Across the Map. *Philosophical Transactions of the Royal Society B: Biological Sciences, 367*(1590), 770–784.

Perreault, C., & Mathew, S. (2012). Dating the Origin of Language Using Phonemic Diversity. *PLoS One, 7*(4), e35289.

Pickrell, J., & Reich, D. (2014). Toward a New History and Geography of Human Genes Informed by Ancient DNA. *Trend in Genetics, 30*(9), 377–389.

Rabaka, R. (2015). *The Negritude Movement: W.E.B. DuBois, Leon Damas, Aimé Césaire, Leopold Senghor, Frantz Fanon, and the Evolution of an Insurgent Idea.* London: Lexington Books.

Raffaele, P. (2007). *Keepers of the Lost Ark?* Smithsonian.com. Retrieved from https://www.smithsonianmag.com/travel/keepers-of-the-lost-ark-179998820/

Syvänne, I. (2017). *Caracalla: A Military Biography.* South Yorkshire: Pen and Sword Military.

The National Archives. *Britain and Slavery.* Retrieved from http://www.nationalarchives.gov.uk/slavery/pdf/britain-and-the-trade.pdf Retrieved 8/7/18

UNESCO. (1990). *Ancient Civilizations of Africa.* London: James Curry Publishing.

Vernus, P., & Yoyotte, J. (2003). *The Book of Pharaohs*. Ithaca, NY: Cornell University.

Zimmer, C. (2016). A Single Migration from Africa Populated the World, Studies Find. *New York Times*. Retrieved from https://www.nytimes.com/2016/09/22/science/ancient-dna-human-history.html

CHAPTER 2

Birth of a Noose: *European Nationalism and Economic Globalism*

Many people look at the history of the world without questioning the etiological factors contributing to the conditions and experiences of those who lived before, during and after the time period under investigation. What was happening in that particular time and space that led to a decision to take a certain action? What outcomes informed subsequent decisions leading to any particular historical context?

According to Washington State Department of Enterprise Services, "The primary goal of using Root Cause Analyses (RCA) is to analyze problems or events to identify: What happened; How it happened; (and) Why it happened ... so that; Actions for preventing recurrence are developed" (Rooney & Vanden-Heuvel, 2004, p. 45). Root causes assess underlying foundations and provide investigators with an analytical tool to construct recommendations, strategies and programs that minimize risk recurrence. Because this approach is not the usual approach taken to explore global involvement in the commencement, maintenance and aftermath of African enslavement, it has in fact repeated itself in a variety of iterations throughout the world.

When historians explore the conditions that led to the rise of Hitler and the National-sozialistische Deutsche Arbeiterpartei (Nazi) party, resulting in the Holocaust, they use a sort of post-mortem RCA. World War I (WWI) began in 1914, lasted over four years and accounted for over 15 million deaths worldwide (Hamilton & Herwig, 2003). When asking the general public: "Why did World war I start?", you are likely to get one of two answers.

© The Author(s) 2019   33
D. E. Grant Jr., *Black Men, Intergenerational Colonialism, and Behavioral Health*, https://doi.org/10.1007/978-3-030-21114-1_2

The first is often: "I don't know" and the second, some iteration of: "The assassination of Archduke Franz Ferdinand and his wife Sophie". For most, simply stating that this assassination occurred is often a sufficient explanation to support the commencement of this bloody and costly war and the atrocities that would follow. RCA approaches, however, force thought processes that see the assassination and the responses to it, not as causal but symptomatic of a pre-existing condition. The assassination was an event that brought to the surface underlying needs that were not being adequately addressed across several domains. These events also serve as significant contributors to the root causes that led to the rise of a leader who would provoke the Jewish Holocaust in a country that had just a half century before been only a collection of small kingdoms and principalities (Hamilton & Herwig, 2003).

The assassination of the Archduke and his wife was carried out in Sarajevo, Bosnia, by Gavrilo Princip after several failed attempts on the same day by other members of the Black Hand, an extreme underground nationalists group to which he belonged. Princip was born in Bosnia into a long tradition of Serbian Christian Orthodoxy. His father was in many ways the equivalent of a Reconstruction Era American share cropper, but in Bosnia. Because one-third of his income was taxed by the Ottoman-ruled Muslim landlords, he was forced to deliver mail and take on other tasks to make money. In 1917, Princip, at 13 years old moved to Sarajevo with his older brother and joined Young Bosnia, an underground revolutionary group of primarily Serbian youth interested in separating Bosnia from the oppressive influence of Austria-Hungary (Hamilton & Herwig, 2003; Watson, 2014).

From the Middle Ages through the thirteenth and fourteenth centuries, Serbians had established several thriving nations, kingdoms and empires recognized by the Romans and the Byzantines of the time, before coming largely under Ottoman rule in the fifteenth and sixteenth centuries. During the first quarter of the nineteenth century, Serbian independence looked imminent. The establishment of the Republic of Serbia and the Hellenic Republic were promising signs, but did not outweigh the extreme oppressive experiences of the millions of ethnic Serbians still under Ottoman and Austro-Hungarian rule living in areas outside of Serbia. To their dismay, after decades of uprisings, the Serbians in Bosnia and Herzegovina, instead of liberation, came under the rule of Austria-Hungary by annexation toward the end of the seventeenth century. This seizure sparked a sense of Serbian nationalism that likely awakened an ancestral link and triggered some historical trauma responses for many involved (Taylor, 2015).

The plot to assassinate the Archduke, heir to the Austro-Hungarian throne, was co-conspired between The Black Hand and the Bosnian government who trained the assassins and provided them with resources including weapons, safe-houses and stealth communication channels. This conspiracy finally gave Austria-Hungary the reason they had been seeking to invade Serbia. They drafted an ultimatum which included demands (intentionally) Serbia was unable/unwilling to meet. When Serbia refused several of the Austro-Hungarian demands, alliances were mobilized: Russia to Serbia and Germany to Austria-Hungary, and war commenced (Hamilton & Herwig, 2003; Taylor, 2015; Watson, 2014).

This assassination and the resultant escalation had been in the making for generations. Once the Ottoman's began to rule these lands, the rights of the Serbians, most of whom were Christian, were all but eliminated. Serbian nobles and intellectuals were murdered, common folk were forced to convert from Christianity to Islam while manual laborers and farmers were forced into conditions of serfdom. Gavrilo Princip's father was one of many ethnic Serbians who fought against the Ottoman Empire's oppressive systems of domination in the seventeenth century. The Bosnian land owners often levied extreme taxes and unjust rules onto the Christian residents occupying the lands they controlled. The intergenerational qualities of unresolved political violence, extreme financial oppression and religious discrimination revolutionized not only at least two generations of Princips, but also the hundreds of Serbian officers and civilians who joined to form organizations like the Black Hand, Young Bosnia and Narodna Odbrana. These groups were often supported by neighboring nations who supplied these rebel groups with armament, weapons and soldiers (Hamilton & Herwig, 2003; Watson, 2014).

In a parallel process, ethnic Serbians successfully maintained a unique cultural heritage while under the severely oppressive feet of several nations (Ottomans, Hapsburgs and Austria-Hungary) across generations. The underlying needs operationalized in the Archduke's assassination were comprised of both a literal and figurative need for liberation after centuries and generations of oppression post-scripting archaeologically supported successful empires. To Princip and his co-conspirators, the Archduke and his wife represented a specific and identifiable obstacle to the actual dismantling of these intergenerationally oppressive holds. They saw the assassination of this heir to the Austro-Hungarian throne as an opportunity for cultural freedom, an end to their institutionalized oppression. The Turkish and Austro-Hungarian oppression of the ethnic Serbians across the diaspora is a root cause to the rise of Hitler (Neiberg, 2017; Taylor, 2015).

Although many see the 1919 Treaty of Versailles as the most important agreement of that time, the many treaties and conventions that dictated the nature of relationships between the world nations might have actually been equally, if not more, influential. Pre-determined relationships, the untracked expiration of existing treaties, leadership transitions and fear all influenced the agreements that informed which countries would support one another during times of war and which would not. Absent those agreements, these conflicts may have never made the international stage, but they did and things escalated quickly as treaties were honored, drawing partners into aggressions that grew largely because the treaty existed. The allyship between the Americans, the Russians, the British and the French proved triumphant against Germany, Austria-Hungary and Italy (Italy had a side agreement with France and would eventually switch sides in the conflict) (Neiberg, 2017).

Germany became a nation in 1871 after the unification of their sovereign states under the rule of Wilhelm I. The Young Bosnian movement actually looked at the German state unification as a model for their work. Their entrepreneurial imperialism, strategic partnerships and militia bolstering set off continental fears in the decades leading up to WWI. Germany saw its WWI defeat as a true national embarrassment, particularly for a nation just developing a uniquely cohesive national identity. They lost over 2 million German soldiers, more than 10% of their European-held territory and all imperial colonies, most of which were in Africa and islands in the South Sea. This set a unique stage for the country throughout the 1920s and 1930s, one whose chronosystem would facilitate one of the world's greatest stains to humanity (Neiberg, 2017).

Hitler was born in Austria in 1889 and showed an early affinity toward German nationalism. Both of his parents died before his 20th birthday, and as a result he spent time as an artist and laborer living between varied homeless shelters in and around Vienna (Rivers, 2015). German nationalism was activated by the early invasions of Napoleon into German states, bringing the question of a German nation-state to the political forefront. The WWI defeat and installation of the subsequent Weimar Republic led to increased and extreme German nationalism characterized by victimization and racial cleansing propaganda, coupled with increasingly anti-social relations with neighboring nations. The Treaty of Versailles left Germany in social shambles, primed for a charismatic leader that would inspire them and embolden their national pride at a time where their sense of national identity was wavering on a shaky foundation. Hitler was appointed chancellor of Germany in 1932 (Rivers, 2015). He used his position, the turbulent German climate, the post-war events and the sentiments of German nationalism to take over full control of the German government. By 1933, the rise of the Nazi Party was complete, they were the only legal political party in Germany and their first leader was in place. Dachau, the first concentration camp, had been established in the state of Bavaria, and the termination of German membership in the League of Nations was solidified. From 1933 through the start of World War II in 1939, Hitler and the Nazi party would implement hundreds of laws that disenfranchised Jewish people. Boycotts of Jewish businesses, exclusion from state service and national organizations, elimination of employment opportunities and restriction from school and university matriculation all culminated in the Nuremberg Laws of 1935, which formally banned marriages between Jewish and non-Jewish Germans. They also stripped German citizenship from those who did not meet the Aryan ethnic identity threshold. By 1838, Aryan zones were created and Jewish people had to carry passports, all while enduring the extreme ethnic violence that was sweeping across Germany. In three short decades, Hitler (d)evolved from a homeless, parentless, teen artist to the sole dictator of Germany responsible for the murder of millions of innocent Jewish people and other individuals he considered undesirable (Davidson, 1997; Hamilton & Herwig, 2003; Rivers, 2015).

The conditions and experiences that led to the Transatlantic Slave Trade are grounded in sixteenth-century European imperialism and informed by centuries of feudalism and warfare. It follows a very similar algorithm to that of the Ottoman and Austro-Hungarian oppression of ethnic Serbians that facilitated the rise of Hitler.

A Curious Quartet

To presume that a nation simply turns into one absent pre-nationalistic development minimizes the true definition of a nation. Nationalism is defined and operationalized in various ways across researchers and disciplines. There are three predominant philosophies and paradigms associated with how it is that nations develop a sense of identity that eventually grows to a broader sense of nationalism, not to be confused with patriotism.

Modernists, Traditionalists and Perennialists tend to occupy these theoretical spaces with a peppering of ideologies from those who identify as Primordialists. Perennialists believe that "nations may have existed for a long time but are not always in the same form", while Primordialists contend that nations are a "timeless phenomenon" (Jensen, 2016). Each of these paradigms is broad in its scope and underserved in its evidence-based support. The dominant Modernists philosophies have historically hosted the highest degrees of prestige across most domains with those of the Traditionalists growing in contemporary research and popularity. Modernists believe that "the nation is a quintessentially modern political phenomenon", while Traditionalists (pre-modern) "believe that nations began to take shape long before the advent of modernity" (Jensen, 2016).

Much of this debate is actually grounded in the question of what makes the nation, "the nation". Modernists often use industrialization, mass media and capitalism as the benchmarks that demarcate a national identity. These variables, due to the recency of their emergence, would easily relegate debates about nationalism to historical contexts that begin only as early as the eighteenth or nineteenth centuries. This severely limits discussions on the historic events that direct a nation's pre- and perinatal development. Some Modernists, in an attempt to honor a wider historical context, incorporate reflections upon the value of communal traditions, collective memories and prevalent symbols of ethnic or cultural affiliations. This is problematic (even with the aforementioned historical addendum), not only for this specific work, but for all related works.

It is widely agreed (among Modernists and Traditionalists) that nationalism is not a primeval concept, yet Azar Gat states that it is "rooted in primordial human sentiments of kin-culture affinity, solidarity and mutual cooperation, evolutionarily engraved in human nature" (Jensen, 2016, p. 31), creating a bridge of change between a develop*ing* nation and a develop*ed* nation. For the following three reasons, the text will adhere to the Traditionalists approach to explore nationalism as one of many root causes for Europe's engagement, leadership and innovations in the Transatlantic Slave Trade; its associated industries, institutions and systems. First, the Modernists approach minimizes the importance of ethnicity and culture in the creation of a nation and its subsequent nationalism. Second, the Modernists' perspectives create a space that effectively absconds the Nation from culpability of infraction due to infancy. Finally, a literature review at the time of this publication demonstrates the

Traditionalists' approach as the dominate one inclusive of the most contemporary evidence-based paradigms (Jensen, 2016).

Most of Europe had been immersed in a series of continental wars between the tenth and the fifteenth century. Issues including, but not limited to violations to shared land governance, egos of nobility, broken treaties, child kings, misogynic throne ascension practices, mental illness, civil war, land domination, famine and deadly plagues where over 30% of the population died all contributed to severe regional instability. Each of these factors served as root causes of European involvement in and leadership of the Transatlantic Slave Trade. To contextualize Europe's involvement, the early histories of four complicit countries are divided across two regional domains which facilitated noteworthy and historically relevant interactions with one another (Green, 2014; White, 2005).

Modern-day Portugal, Spain, England and France are four of the most important European nations responsible for the initiation and proliferation of Africa's (and other indigenous lands of color) colonization and the Earth's most insidious slave trade. The intertwined histories of England and France in the west differ from those of modern-day Spain and Portugal on the Iberian Peninsula to the south east. Their histories occurred independently but juxtaposed by time and interconnected by context resulting in a cacophonous synergy. One where the removal and commodification of people and resources was government and religiously sanctioned (Green, 2014; White, 2005).

The ecological environments in which history occurs create conditions that generate a myriad of potential responses, some pro-social, some anti-social, very few are ever neutral. The varied stages of development that a nation moves through within these environments birth the national sentiment, set the national norms and operationalize a citizenry's patriotic tone. There are a very specific set of circumstances that coalesced to inform Europe's decision to lead the world in the endorsement and participation in an institutionalized industry that would change the course and trajectory of every continent on Earth. European imperialism and colonialism, the institutionalization of slavery, the commencement of the Transatlantic Slave Trade and the industries they shaped birthed the economic infrastructure that directly catalyzed global industrialization and each continent's Industrial Revolution and Moral Devolution.

Portugal and Castile (currently Spain) represent ground zero of what would become one of the most protracted global industries, the Transatlantic Slave Trade. Portugal was the first European player in the

Transatlantic Slave Trade and is identified as a significant world power by the end of the fifteenth century. They shared a unique relationship with Spain that many historians describe as the key to their downfall as a world power broker. The County of Portugal developed just before the start of the tenth century and grew in size and importance relatively quickly. The Kingdom of Portugal was established after a local civil war distracted enemies allowing Portugal's Count to expand their geographic reach of power by joining two counties. Success in the Battle of Sao Mamede in 1128 marks Portugal's nationhood. Its first documented king, Afonso Henriques, would be recognized in 1139. He would go on to annex surrounding lands from the Moors, almost doubling the kingdom's land mass and creating stability for an independent monarchy that would gain regional and international notoriety (Green, 2014; Kelsey, 2003; Thomas, 2014).

The kingdom of Castile had a long history of union and disunion with the kingdom of León during European medieval history. Like the developmental stages of other nations—and people—Castile was at an early stage wrought with civil wars, familial disputes, assassinations and land annexations. This budding nation's development would reach adolescence in the late fifteenth century when Ferdinand II of Aragon married Queen Isabella I of Castile. Ferdinand became the King of Castile, by marriage, a noble status that was not just ceremonial. In 1479, Ferdinand would ascend as king of Aragon after his fathers' death, inheriting the territories of Aragon and uniting them with the crown of Castile to become one body politic, España (Spain). Although many municipal concerns remained localized, they would centralize their noble power and possessions to successfully move the last of the Moors out of the region ending the Reconquista and reinstating Catholic rule over the Iberian Peninsula after centuries of Muslim domination (Kelsey, 2003; Thomas, 2014).

Throughout the entirety of the fourteenth and fifteenth centuries, England and France were largely at war with one another. In 1066, the Duke of Normandy—a feudal French fief holder—gained control of the English throne. This led to generations of English rulers born from French lineage often already in possession of French territory. As a result, English royalty had long held legal claims to French territories, which at several points in history were greater in size than the French lands actually ruled by the French. This, for obvious reasons, was a significant threat to the French kings who would make consistent attempts to dismantle English control and influence within the country. When the English attempted to expand their reach to the French throne due to an apparently unforeseen hiccup in the royal business continuity plan, tensions built and former concessions met their pending breach. This catalyzed eminent territorial disputes that had been brewing for generations and that would last for even more generations.

Most medieval European municipalities thrived during the time prior to the Hundred Years War. France had been the most dominant power in Western Europe, but the English army consistently demonstrated themselves as a force to be reckoned with during the Hundred Years War beginning in 1337. Battles would ensue across the continent. Land and territory would move from French to English and back again. Only 10 years after the start of the war, the continent would fall epidemically ill as a result of the bubonic plague. Arriving along the "Silk Road"—a trading route connecting Central Asia to Europe through the Middle East—the plague would kill over 30% of the continents population (20 million people) and millions more worldwide. The devastation of the plague juxtaposed to the war at hand created a significant economic crisis. Consistent with most pandemics and multi-national wars that occur simultaneously, individuals at the lowest end of the socio-economic strata are disproportionately impacted. In medieval Europe, these were the peasants and serfs (derived from Latin *servus* meaning slave), those bound to the land of the manorial society and the Lord of the fief (Green, 2014; White, 2005).

The Peasants' Revolt of 1381 was a direct response to the chronosystem created by each of these medieval events. The Bubonic Plague devastated communities of peasants and serfs in urban and rural areas of both England and France. England, under great financial distress, began to levy taxes on the poor to recoup finances lost during the Hundred Years War. They collected poll taxes, fixed wages and barred laborers from raising their rates. The rebels descended on London burning buildings and killing royal government officials until their demands were met. By the end of the revolt, the rebels had secured a reduction in taxation and the abolition of serfdom, a common form of forced labor throughout feudal Europe. This revolt empowered Europe's underclass momentarily and rendered the royal government reluctant (at best) to levy any additional taxes against the poor to pay for the remainder of the war. It would be months of beheadings and executions before the royal government would be able to fully suppress the uprisings. When the royal government regained control, they revoked most all agreements made with the rebels during the revolt and reinstated the institution of serfdom (Green, 2014; White, 2005).

Most of the entire Hundred Years War was fought on French soil, decimating its infrastructure and population. Although the English still held Paris, in 1429 Joan of Arc led a French brigade to the Battle of Orleans and effectively forced the English militia to retreat back across the Loire River, reigniting the French spirit. The Hundred Years War ended without official treaty or agreement in 1453 when France reclaimed the hotly debated territory of Gascony during the Battle of Castillon. France had gained much of its territory back, and England conceded maintaining control only over Calais. England rejected all things French, including the language which had been widely spoken in England since the mid-eleventh century, painting the future of their self-definition and relationship between one another (Green, 2014; White, 2005).

As a result of the Hundred Years War, The Bubonic Plague and the European Peasants' Revolution, both England and France lost large portions of their populations and wealth. French cities and towns had been ravished by looting, arson and the murders of thousands of civilians. Population had decreased dramatically, serfs escaped the land to which they were bound, trade declined increasing the cost of goods and peasants continued to revolt in both France and England. England would find themselves immersed in two more conflict-ridden decades with the start of The War of the Roses, a civil war for the English throne commencing almost immediately following the end of the Hundred Years War. This marked the end of European feudalism, the manorial system, serfdom and medieval times overall. Both countries had matured and evolved into their nationalistic heritages.

Contemporary research evidences the severe toll that is taken on the citizenry of a geographic area immersed in generations of warfare. Now that the wars were over, what was the country and its citizens to do with all this residual trauma, excess time and newly available cognitive energy? Due to the centuries that separate contemporary research from the experiences of old Europe, one cannot presume to fully generalize outcomes across these times. One can, however, based on the neurological and behavioral responses specifically related to these events, deduce that several factors were highly likely and even ever-present.

Those who were "drafted" to fight for the English and French crowns in battles across generations were more often than not poor people and serfs. Once the wars were over, they were able to tend to their farms, perhaps catch up on rents due to landlords and maybe spend time with family. Some even took time to mourn the losses of loved ones and to re-regulate their lives to the new normal. Generations of trauma are sure to have significantly influenced those who likely suffered the greatest losses. Research on the Community Loss Index demonstrates that chronic stress and loss results in a collective impact on the mind and body that can manifest itself in poor health and social outcomes in both the community and individual context. These outcomes negatively influence the community's ability to function at optimal levels. Not only do these factors impact health and social outcomes, they can also "heighten individuals' perceptions of risk, shatter their basic assumptions about safety and protection and undermine their sense of trust and place" (Abramovitz & Albrecht, 2013, p. 679).

The behaviors and practices of the nobility also looked different during this post-war era. They too surely suffered significant loss while the same intergenerational traumas of a war-torn century painted their existence. Although both these groups experienced the exact same environmental stimuli, the socio-culture space they occupied during the experience renders their loss and responses to these losses different across several domains. During war, the affairs, finances and families of nobility were left largely intact due to the structure of the European class (caste) system of the time. It is widely speculated that the period of over-indulgence and conspicuous consumption following the wars demonstrates the mental and behavioral framework of the English nobility during this short lived time of peace. Some even believe that peace time was the actual antithesis to the existence of nobility given the identity structure on which nobility is built, one that emphasizes the value of paid homage, excellence in battle, annexation of territory and increased wealth. England, as a result, would soon see its nobility engaged in hunting, hawking and banqueting, all uncommon activities heretofore.

As a result, these nation's military tactics became more advanced, they were more politically savvy and most noteworthy, citizens of each country began to crystallize a new sense of cohesive national identity (Wilde, 2018). One of the most critical points in the history of any country is when evidence of a unified countrywide identity first surfaces. Research demonstrates that people who experience events and conditions imbued with strife and stress together have a high propensity for increased group cohesion and the adoption of a group identity. For both France and England: ending the war, surviving the plague and empowering the peasant class all provided very specific experiences that would inform their next steps.

David Bell defines nationalism as "a conscious political programme aimed at the construction of a nation where one didn't exist" (Jensen, 2016, p. 71) which is separate from that of national identity, patriotism or pride. Hass (Hass, 1986) defined nationalism as "… the convergence of territorial and political loyalty irrespective of competing foci of affiliation, such as kinship, profession, religion, economic interest, race, or even language" (Hass, 1986, p. 709). This definition provides a context that uniquely unites many people living within a particular geographic boundary inside a specific chronosystemic space. Although unity tends to connote a heterogeneity of thought and a utopian system of equality, it is used here to demonstrate a strong, and admittedly often contentious, relationship between people existing at different ends of the class continuum in these same spaces of time. In 1787, the enslaved Black American man fought for American Independence along the same lines of allegiance as the White American man. The White American Revolutionary War soldier was, at best, a supporter and benefactor of the enslavement of Black Americans and at worst an active participant in the institution. Although the perspectives of each soldier differ about as much as is possible, each engages in one of the most noteworthy nationalistic efforts offered to lay folk.

When a nation has "liberated itself from older political and social formations, the advancement to a new spirit of nationhood at a higher level" (Jensen, 2016, p. 48) will move the nation to the development of a more comprehensive and holistic sense of self. Once the nation begins to establish itself, it is thought to go through a sort of a second phase of nation-building, much aligned to the stages of human psychosocial and psychosexual development as described by Erik Erikson and Sigmund Freud, respectively. In each stage of these models, both the individual and the nation find themselves immersed in events that influence and inform development. The values that are held closest, the varied threat responses, the way love, support and admiration is received and the way difference is (dis)engaged are each critical factors that demonstrate how both the individual and the nation develop across its lifespan. It is no coincidence that both the individual and the nation grow in parallel processes along a similar developmental framework: No People, No Nation.

Developmentalists describe adolescence as a time period by which a person moves from being a child to a young adult. During this time, noteworthy cognitive, biological and socio-cultural factors shape outcomes that operationalize themselves throughout the entirety of the adult lifespan. The experiences of adolescence are all informed by the individuals' childhood and pre-natal experiences, laying the groundwork for this very important transitional period. Studies on Adverse Childhood Experiences (ACE's) unambiguously identify childhood traumas as complicit in the development of affective disorders, hallucinations, psychosis and anti-social behaviors in teens and adults (Whitfield, Dube, Felitti, & Anda, 2005). Chronologically, humans experience adolescence from puberty through their mid-20s, and some researchers have moved that mark as far out as 25. Adolescence is marked by an ability to think in the abstract, the development of a wider perspective beyond "the self", a capacity for metacognition and introspection and the propensity to take risks. Each of these factors contributes to adolescences' primary goal, the development of identity (White, 2005).

By the end of the fifteenth century, Spain, Portugal, England and France had all reached very critical places in their nationalistic development. As it relates to their national identity (compared to collections of nation-states), both Spain and Portugal had reached adolescence while England and France were experiencing pre-pubescent angsts. By the start of the sixteenth century, each nation would find itself in the throes of adolescence and identity formation, Spain and Portugal in late adolescents and France and England in the early stages. The studies of organic chemistry and molecular biology exist to understand the nature, structure and function of those non-living molecules that sustain the human body's functions and responses to the environment. These disciplines have generated a rich body of knowledge that explains disease, neurological functioning, nutrition and reproduction among other things. In the same ways that studies on the structure and function of molecules in the human body contribute to the developmental functions and behaviors of the human, studies on the microsystemic events and conditions of the people in a nation contribute great knowledge to the development of that nation and its national identity.

The development of both humans and nations is based upon actors and outcomes, each of which is influenced by the space in which the development occurs while simultaneously impacting that space. The events that Europe experienced across the centuries marked these nations' individual and collective experiences. These nation-states began to cultivate nationalism similarly to how individuals develop self-identity and esteem. In the same way high ACE scores influence a child's trajectory into adolescence and adulthood, a nation's early experiences inform their next steps of development toward that of nationhood. In this case, their histories of adverse and propitious geographic experiences left each nation, in early adolescence, with a need to expand its reach, influence and wealth beyond its geographic borders. These developmental needs would dominate each nation's entry into the sixteenth century and entrepreneurial colonial development.

The decision to establish colonies is one that nations in varying stages of development make using (consciously or not) the experiences that painted its earlier development. The Portuguese, Spanish, English and French were by no means the first nations to institute the use of colonial lands, and in fact the Greeks and Romans had done it for generations before. An analysis of etiological factors that lead to a nation's colonialistic instinct is retrospectively predictive of how the colony was to be populated and nurtured, the levels of religious restrictiveness and how, if at all, it would be deliberately situated for the financial gain of the motherland.

Greece and Rome established colonies away from their homelands in ways that appear to have arisen from need. The historical record seems to support two ways ancient colonies were established. In one scenario, the motherlands of Greece, as a result of shared borders with hostile neighbors, were unable to simply expand the lands on which they inhabited. When populations grew to a capacity beyond which the motherland could support, "a part of them were sent in quest of a new habitation in some remote and distant part of the world" (Smith, 1994, p. 249). In a second, slightly more complex scenario, the impoverished Romans were left with no other options but to identify new lands on which to live. In *The Wealth of Nations*, Adam Smith describes how ancient Roman societies were fully reliant upon the labor of the enslaved in that,

> a poor freeman had had little chance of being employed as a farmer or labourer. All trades and manufactures too, even the retail trade, were carried on by the slaves of the rich for the benefit of their masters, whose wealth, authority and protection made it difficult for a poor freeman to maintain competition against them. (Smith, 1994, p. 600)

The rich were neither willing to part with their land or their slaves. This created a unique dynamic ripe for the uprising of the poor. To remedy this concern and quell uprisings, the republic would create an opportunity for the development of colonies on lands familiar to the mother city. Through this effort, Rome both provided satisfaction to its poorest residents and established influential strongholds for itself in geographic proximal spaces whose allegiance might have otherwise been uncertain. In each scenario, the motivation for Greek and Roman colonial development was clear and highly grounded in necessity at best and utility at worst. "The establishment of the European colonies in America and the West Indies arose from no necessity; and though the utility which has resulted from them has been very great, it (the decision to colonize) is not altogether so clear and evident" (Smith, 1994, p. 601).

Global Imperialism and European Colonialism

European imperialism and global colonization practices serve as a sort of proclamation emanating from nationalistic histories. Imperialism represents a nation's philosophy of power and domination as a tool to extend its influence onto foreign entities through land acquisition and military maneuvers. Colonialism—imperialisms counterpart—is the practice of annexing another country for political control. It often involves occupying the land with workers and settlers and subsequently exploiting its natural resources for economic and political gain. Imperialism was the paradigmatic guiding light of European Colonialisms' journey across the globe. When Colonialism met the Trans-African Slave Trade, he was enamored and intrigued. It wasn't long before they united to take the pre-existing system of capitalism to a new height.

"As the center of global capitalism, Europe not only had control of the world market, but it was also able to impose its colonial dominance over all the regions and populations of the planet, incorporating them into its world-system and its specific model of power" (Quijano & Ennis, 2000, p. 540). Capitalism can be traced back to the early sixteenth century and is thought to be the offspring of mercantilism and the grand child of feudalism. Immanuel Wallerstein developed the World Systems Analysis in the 1970s and describes the three historical systems that have existed across the lifespan of the modern human. The mini-systems are those that we often reflect upon with indigenous populations' historic livelihood sustained through the formation of bands, chiefdoms and tribes. According to Wallerstein, the mini-system evolved into one world-system predicated on a level of political homogeneity, which would then evolve into our contemporary poly-political global economy. World Systems Theory takes a high level look at global history and patterns of social change by dividing international regions of labor into three categories, placing emphasis on the "world-system" as the primary actor when assessing for outcomes. This is—as compared to other models that focus on individual nations, countries and municipalities—the key influencing factor. Some who ascribe to this analysis go as far to say that no country has an economy, but that they are all a part of a larger world economy (Wallerstein, 2004).

Core Nations hold wealth and wield power as the labor force (en masse) focuses on higher-order operating skills and efforts that require a higher degree of capital for execution. They operate effectively absent outside control and have significant influence on other nations, both peer and non-core. Semi-peripheral nations have a smaller influence on the world's economy, are less involved in non-regional international trade and are primarily responsible for the provision of services in the grand scheme of this theoretical framework. Spain and Portugal were further into their national development than France and England by the end of the fifteenth century. They, as a result of several important factors, developed national identities of dominance that promoted and inspired a practice of exploration to oppress, conquer and "civilize". "(F)or people who experience strong feelings of national superiority, the preferred outcomes are domination over other nations and the policing of the nation's symbolic boundaries against undesirable others" (Bonikowski, 2016, p. 430).

There were several factors that led Europe to believe they could, and even more disturbingly *would*, create an institution around the conquering of diverse lands inhabited by phenotypically analogous people. In 2009, researchers discovered Finca Clavijo, the oldest known of the cemeteries for enslaved Africans on the Atlantic sea coast. It was situated next to an ancient sugar plantation in Santa Maria de Guia, on the Canary Islands. Researchers and archaeologists conducted DNA analysis, isotopic radiocarbon dating and skeletal marker assessments of physical activity on the remains of the 14 people found (Santana et al., 2016). This 2016 study published in the Journal of Physical Anthropology confirms that the individuals lived during the fifteenth and seventeenth centuries, and all died in their 20s. Mitochondrial DNA analysis traces their lineage to North and Sub-Saharan Africa while indicators of physical activity show a pattern of labor involving high levels of exertion similar to those of remains found on South Carolinian plantations of the eighteenth and nineteenth centuries. The cemetery also provided evidence of non-Christian customs, traditions and funerary practices well into the seventeenth century, challenging some theories of early spiritual and cultural genocide (Santana et al., 2016).

The Canary Islands, an archipelago just off the coast of Morocco, was described as "stepping stones into the Atlantic" by Felipe Fernández-Armesto (Berquist Soule, 2017). Portugal made their first mission to the islands in 1341 and came back with goods and a small number of enslaved natives. Although the Italians, Castilians and Moroccans had reached and even inhabited the islands across the thirteenth and fourteenth centuries, Portugal's 1341 religiously inspired militaristic delegation would be one of many actions that provided Europe with evidence to support their genocidal imperialistic urges.

In 1343, Castile launched a mission to these same islands. Ignoring Portugal's prior undertaking, the Castilians claimed the group of islands as their own. They proceeded to set up missions to convert the natives to Christianity. As the presence of the Catholic Church increased on the archipelago, so did that of sailors, pirates, slavers and other traders. In 1402, Castile launched its first military operative on the islands. Gaining control of the Canary Islands meant access to slave labor and one step closer to the gold of Guinea, what Africa was known as at this time in Europe.

During the fifteenth century (long before and long after), the papacy of the Roman Catholic Church not only regulated religious doctrine and moral code, they were also routinely invited to mediate political clashes, like land disputes between different kingdoms, the distribution of wealth and the enslavement of people. In the early years of Atlantic exploration, both Portugal and Castile were competing for claims of African territory. If these pursuits were a Hollywood film, the Catholic Church would function as screenwriter, director, producer, cinematographer and editor.

The early perspective of the Catholic church was able to effectively embrace a notable, but thin division of church and state. In the thirteenth century, Pope Innocent IV contended that the jurisdiction of the church was over the spirituality of humans (Christians and others), and individuals being guided by their own municipal laws were not in violation of Catholic doctrine. According to Pope Innocent IV, not only were they not violating natural law, "invading their territory, enslaving them, and seizing their lands was not sanctioned" (Berquist Soule, 2017, p. 21). This meant that the activities on the Canaries were in fact a direct violation of the church's orders, orders that would soon change.

Apostolatus officium (1403) was a Papal Bull from Pope Benedict VII that moved the efforts in Canaries to what has been shown to have been a full on Christian Crusade. The identity of native islanders was firmly and strategically crystallized to heathens, infidels and heretics, justifying a religious war. Although there were limits to Benedict's bull regarding the enslavement of islanders who had converted to Christianity, Portuguese and Castilian slave raids, captures and kidnapping ran virally across the entire archipelago. This environment was not conducive to the goals (explicit and implicit) of the Castilians and Portuguese. This chaos and dissatisfaction incited further papal involvement resulting in Pope Eugenius IV's bull, *Creator omnium*, which doubled down on Innocents position and even threatened excommunication for "one and all who attempt to capture or sell or subject to slavery [any] baptized residents of the Canary Islands" (Berquist Soule, 2017, p. 21).

Pope Nicholas V took a more decisive stance on the African land and its people. Pope Nicholas V issued both the *Dum Diversas* in 1452 and the *Romanus Pontifex* in 1455. France and England were still recovering from The Hundred Years War as Portugal was beginning their imperialistic reign of terror shrouded in a Christian invisibility cloak. At the request of Portugal's Christian king Afonso V, Pope Nicholas V, in 1452, granted him with "Apostolic Authority, full and free permission to invade, search out, capture, and subjugate the Saracens and pagans and any other unbelievers and enemies of Christ wherever they may be … and reduce their persons into perpetual servitude" (Adiele, 2017, p. 313). In *Romanus Pontifex* (1455), Pope Nicholas V writes:

> … if we bestow suitable favors and special graces on those Catholic kings and princes, who, like athletes and intrepid champions of the Christian faith, as we know by the evidence of facts, not only restrain the savages excesses of the Saracens and of other infidels, enemies of the Christian name, but also for the defense and increase of the faith vanquish them and their kingdoms and habitations, though situated in the remotest parts unknown to us. (Davenport, 2004, p. 21)

These papal bulls (retracted in 1807) effectively provided the country of Portugal with three major gifts: A monopoly on trade and commerce in all new areas explored on the African continent, the legal right to raid foreign ships in those territories and the blessing of the Roman Catholic Church to enslave Africans, Moors and Saracens (Arabs) (Adiele, 2017).

The efforts of the Catholic Church were being consistently violated, so much so that it wouldn't be unreasonable that mixed messages were being generated and delivered to those with proverbial and literal "boots on the ground". *Pastor bonus* was a papal bull issued by Pope Pius II in 1462 which, again, threatened excommunication for those violating the laws of The Church. He demanded that their freedom be restored and their belongings returned immediately. Queen Isabella and King Ferdinand of Castile would take an opportunity to operationalize The Church's unambiguous order in 1477 when Fernand Peraza, charged with overseeing Canarian operations on the island of Gomera, returned with 1000 captured natives from Gomera prepared for sale in the Southern Spanish slave markets. Months after their arrival, the Castilian Crown released the natives and returned them to the Canaries. Unfortunately, these captives would return to their homeland under severe suppression from the Spanish, specifically Peraza, the Christian overseer tasked with supporting their spiritual conversion (Adiele, 2017; Berquist Soule, 2017; Kelsey, 2003).

As with many colonially oppressed indigenous communities, their empowerment resulted in their extinction. Overwhelmed and overworked by Peraza, the Gomeros would soon rise up against the Spanish subjugation and kill their overseer. This created a layer of complexity which promoted further and more intense exploration of the islands under the guise of Christianity. It appeared that the Spanish Crown's imperialistic worldview was forming atop a foundation of duality bordering hypocrisy. Some native people on lands they colonized were given the option to convert to Christianity, some did and some didn't. Those who converted were oftentimes still sold into the Andalusian slave markets, those who didn't were automatically enslaved. There was, however, another group of native people, those for whom a choice to accept or reject Christianity was never granted. These indigenous people were simply conquered and enslaved on sight. The Gomeros and the Guanches were both conquered on different parts of the archipelago and in less than one generation were effectively wiped from the historic record, although evidence of their ancestral DNA can still be found on the islands. The Treaty of Alcaçovas (1479) would finally put to rest the centuries of battle between Portugal and Castile regarding the fate of the Canary Islands. This treaty would also serve as an initial blueprint for the Transatlantic Slave Trade that would follow.

The Age of Discovery: Architects of an Institution

An institution is defined as an established set of laws, customs or practices. Not all institutions cover each of these defining characteristics but many do. The institution of slavery is one of them, one that meets the definition across a literal global framework of key players, stakeholders, victims and survivors. The capture, purchase and enslavement of Black and African people was protected under several established laws throughout several European countries. It became customary and routine for families to not only hold enslaved Black and African people as their property but to publically dismantle their characters and spirits physically and psychologically. Finally, the practices of capturing Africans, enslaving Black people and sustaining the plantation economy were deliberately documented practices that resulted in a set of standard operating procedures for the successful maintenance of the institution (Adiele, 2017; Berquist Soule, 2017; Kelsey, 2003).

It is common knowledge that the practice of enslaving people has existed in several forms throughout the history of the world. Europe, Asia, the Middle East and Africa had all engaged in the enslavement of people across generations. Whether they were spoils of war, purchased for service or the result of a kingdoms merger, they were all held captive against their individual and collective wills. The Roman military regularly captured thousands of slaves during battles. At the end of the fourteenth century, Spanish slave markets provided an assorted population of Moors, Greeks, Orthodox Christians, Canary Islanders, Black Africans, Circassians, Russians and Tartars for purchase. England's rural agricultural communities depended on serfs and slaves. After the Bubonic Plague, Europe saw a severe shortage in labor due to the plague's disproportionately fatal impact on the poor. As a result, they began to import enslaved people from all over Europe, the Middle East and Northern Africa (Berquist Soule, 2017).

Prince Henry, Queen Isabella, King Ferdinand and Christopher Columbus were all early adopters in the positioning of the European nations to proactively orchestrate the genocidal imperialistic practices on which globalization and its economy would be built. It is rarely possible to gain post-mortem intention to historic motivation. This current exploration attends to that reality by simply presenting queries for the exploration of human existentialism.

The Portuguese were visionaries among fifteenth-century ship building circles. Prior to their innovations, most ships were ill fitted for long journeys over stormy waters. Many countries experienced extreme tragedy on the sea. They often underestimated its fortitude and over-estimated their own ingenuity. Prince Henry "the Navigator" would change the course of history for this small European country, its neighbors and three other continents. Prince Henry's father was Portugal's king, and his mother was the sister of England's king. Born in 1394, he is widely known for his patrimonial role in ushering Europe into what is now known as The Age of Discovery. He was instrumental in Portugal's first African occupation: Ceuta which was in Morocco just across the Strait of Gibraltar. This occupation facilitated the birth of this young Princes' aspirations which would then be catalyzed by a stream of significant events. Prince Henry created nautical and navigational schools and facilitated the development of one of the most successful maritime industries in all of Europe. Through his work, the Portuguese: refined navigation tools, developed multi-disciplinary nautical teams, mastered cartography and combined best practices in ship building and naval architecture to create the caravels and the naus. These sailing ships were able to maneuver through treacherous sea storms over many miles and across months at a time (Kelsey, 2003; Thomas, 2014). Were his drive, curiosity and innovation just markers and benchmarks of a young Princes' efforts to self-actualize? Although he rarely participated directly in the colonial and imperial expeditions across the Atlantic, he surely knew what the expertise he created was being used for, but did he care?

Queen Isabella and King Ferdinand, both born of royal blood (they were first cousins), married one another at 18 and 17, respectively. From the start of their reign, they exercised a paradigm of domination grounded on the creation of a monolithic, nationalistic Christian society. Others who were forced to convert (those who converted voluntarily often did so under the threat of death or expulsion) to Christianity from Islam or Judaism were arbitrarily recognized if at all. Their royal power and specific lens synergized in the Edict of Expulsion and Spanish Inquisition, persecuting, executing and expelling thousands of Castilian and Aragonian Muslims and Jews. They financed the exploration of the Atlantic and endorsed the genocide of native people across several continents in the name of Christianity. The Pope would grant them the title of the "Catholic Monarchs", due in part to their vigilant defense of Christendom (Adiele, 2017). Were Queen Isabella and King Ferdinand's protection and expansion of Christianity demonstrative of a disarmingly strong faith in Christ and dedication to God and the papacy or was it connected to the spoils associated with the advancement of this specific agenda?

Christopher Columbus was born in 1451 in Genoa (now a part of Italy) and grew up in Savona, a major Italian seaport. Today, his dad Domenico would be considered a lower middle-class entrepreneur of sorts. Although he was a third-generation weaver, he also ran several shops and small businesses. He never met with great financial success, incentivizing his sons to break the weaving tradition and head for the seas. Columbus, eager to move from his economic station, became a skilled navigator and experienced international trader. He learned several languages and read a broad array of literature on history, astronomy and geography; he was also known to frequently quote the Bible.

Imperialism was a growing theme of expansion for Castile and Portugal. Columbus had presented several very ambitious exploration plans to the thrones of Castile, Portugal and Rome. All were declined. He was tenacious in his search for the opportunity to gain wealth and influence, an opportunity finally granted by King Ferdinand and Queen Isabella. Columbus brokered a deal known as the Capitulations of Santa Fe where he would be appointed Viceroy and Governor of all lands he colonized for The Catholic Monarchy; in addition, he would get a percentage of all commercial profits from the new colonies (Esposito, 2015; Thomas, 2014). Was Columbus so desperately driven to change the social status into which he was born that he would use his talents for cultural extermination? Would he engage in the literal and figurative genocides of generations to move the fate of himself and his two sons? What might he have been reflecting upon as he wiped the existence of entire cultures of people from the historic record?

One may never know if these individuals had foresight into knowledge of or even intentionality in what would be their longest-lived legacies as the architects of the Trans-African Slave Trade. After the capture of Ceuta, the Portuguese began to explore further and farther south. Their new ships afforded them opportunities that had not ever before existed. Cape Bojador, a small peninsula on the northwestern Saharan coast, had been the most distant point on the continent of Africa that Europeans had accessed. By 1441, Prince Henry was sending groups of traders and explorers beyond Cape Bojador to explore more of Africa and to find a direct maritime route to the gold-producing regions of sub-Saharan West Africa. By 1444, they had circumvented the Muslim and Ottoman land-based trade route and made their way past the southern portion of the Saharan Desert, creating a sea-based trade route to Africa. In 1445, they had established a trading fort at The Bay of Arguin just off the coast of what is today Mauritania where they traded ivory, grain, copper and African people. Throughout the remainder of the fifteenth century, the Portuguese would explore more and more of the West African coastline. In addition to the creation of continental forts, they also found the Atlantic islands of Cape Verde, São Tomé and Príncipe. They colonized these allegedly uninhabited islands and would later use them as collection points for enslaved African captives and commodities heading to the Americas and back to the Iberian Peninsula. The Crown of Castile was paying close attention to the Portuguese exploration and sought protection over the possessions they had acquired. The only way to ensure that a meaningful compromise would be attained was to seek the support of the Catholic Church. The Roman Catholic Church would be one of the first businesses, along with the kingdoms of Portugal and Spain, to gain great wealth as a result of the colonization of Western Africa and the institution of slavery. Much of the early blood money of the slave trade went to support the training, education and institutions dedicated to uplift Catholic and Jesuit priests, seminarians, missionaries and congregants (Adiele, 2017; Thomas, 2014).

Ecological imperialism and the Columbian Exchange: Before the arrival of the colonists, the Americas and its indigenous people had never been exposed to the epidemic-inducing bacteria and viruses brought over from Europe. Diseases like small pox, measles, influenza, tuberculosis, cholera, pneumonia and hepatitis wiped natives out by the droves forcing the land into poverty as their forced labor pool was depleted. Well over 60% of the entire hemisphere died as a result of what would come to be known as "The Columbian Exchange" built on Spanish cruelty and disease (Esposito, 2015; Thomas, 2014).

In the sixteenth and seventeenth centuries, England created an ecosystem supportive of malaria breakouts. By demanding the draining of swamp lands for farming, Queen Elizabeth I would trigger the second deadly epidemic their people would see across two centuries. Drained swamp land remained moist and perfect for farming. It was also perfect breeding ground for the Anopheles mosquitoes that carried the deadly virus. With no sea water to wash out the larvae, the mosquitoes had opportunities to complete its life cycle in places it had not been able to before. These marshlands in southern and southeastern England would experience exponential population declines while other areas thrived. As malaria spread from the marshlands to other areas in England, it also made its way to the North American colonies (Berquist Soule, 2017).

By the seventeenth century, ships were traveling relatively frequently back and forth between the "New World" (which wasn't new since generations of people were already there) and English ports where malaria was claiming victims at a shocking rate. Over half of all the new settlers in the English colonies on North America came from what became known as "the Malaria Belt" (Mann, 2014). Malaria likely made its way to the Americas in the early seventeenth century by both colonists who arrived in Jamestown, along Virginia's Chesapeake Bay from the infected ports of Europe, and enslaved African captives. From 1606 through 1612, costal Virginia was experiencing a severe drought. The streams and brooks that usually flowed into the Chesapeake quickly evaporated until they were mere standing pools of stagnant water. This combined with the warmth and humidity of the North American colonial South created a climate perfectly situated for both the life cycle of the Anopheles mosquito and the spread of the deadly disease it carried. Of the small group of English settlers who first arrived to settle in Jamestown in 1607, we know the birth places of just 59 of them. Of that 59, 37 arrived from malaria-infected English counties (Esposito, 2015; Thomas, 2014).

English investors became increasingly anxious after the failure of New Edinburgh, a proposed Scottish colony in modern-day Panama. The people of Scotland invested upward of 50% of their countries' liquid assets to the development of this colony which would control commerce between the Atlantic and Pacific oceans. A significant contributor to the downfall of New Edinburgh was death from disease: malaria, yellow fever and dysentery specifically. Of the first group of Scottish settlers, over 70% died from disease and infection, the others returned to Scotland as over a thousand new settlers headed for the Central American colony with the potential to secure a monopoly on trade between Asia and Europe. The vast majority of this second group would also fall fatally to these ravishing diseases. The few who were able to survive would flee Panama for Scotland after less than one year (Esposito, 2015; Thomas, 2014).

New Edinburgh was a complete disaster, sparking riots in Scotland and panic in England. Although England and Scotland were separate nations, they shared a monarch (along with Wales) after the death of Queen Elizabeth I and adoption of the Union of Crowns. As Scotland burned with riotous panic, its legislative body and elite were in need of a return on their investment. England agreed to cover the financial ramifications of colonial failure under the Acts of Union which would also result in the joining of Scotland with England to birth Great Britain. When Virginia began to foreshadow the same symptoms of colonial death at the infantile stage of development, a decision had to be made to ensure the success of the colonies (Baptiste, 2015; Thomas, 2014).

As malaria made its way around the Atlantic coastal colonies in the southern portions of North America, colonists and Parliament were faced with an important decision. In order to effectively increase their output, the importation of labor was necessary. Models for both slavery and indentured servitude had been well established throughout the history of the "Old World", and the "New World" (managed by Old World guards) needed to choose the labor force to build their new lands (Baptiste, 2015; Thomas, 2014).

Sickle Cell Anemia is a condition that almost exclusively impacts individuals of African descent across the diaspora living in places other than the African continent, particularly in America. Sickle Cell Anemia provides a genetic anthropological foot print explaining the geo-biological selectivity of the enslaved African. Although malaria is known to have existed millennia ago, its first known record in the Americas coincides with European colonialism. Abnormalities of blood cell structure (like sickle cell) are the most well-known and studied genetic resistances to malaria (Esposito, 2015). Those who acquired resistance as a result of exposure represent the second most prevalent group of people least like to ever acquire the virus. Research further demonstrates that a sort of enhanced immunity results from exposure to the virus for those who already have one of the pre-existing blood cell abnormalities, hugely increasing survivability in areas where death from malaria was more likely than not (Esposito, 2015).

The colonists were certainly no experts at the epidemiology of malaria and yellow fever, but it didn't take long for them to implement ecological protective factors that reduced their risk of death from the disease. In 1892, R.Q. Mallard reflects "the summer months were spent by the White families in what was known as 'summer retreats', or villages located out in the pine forests; the return to the plantation was not considered safe until a killing frost had fallen". When they returned to their plantations in the autumn and winter months, their enslaved Africans had survived the dangers of malaria and yellow fever (Mallard, 1892).

Imperialism, colonialism, religiosity, epidemiology and nobility all contributed to the growth and prosperity of Britain's colonial empire in the Americas. The need for a labor source to support the development of the colonies just to meet the promise of imperialistic wealth was clear. What became even more clear during this process was the "type" of labor force that would become preferential for colonial growth, development and success. Evidence demonstrates that the mass enslavement of Africans would have still likely happened absent the devastation of European and native populations by malaria, small pox and yellow fever. It is critical to note that during this time, when the speed with which the colonies grew hastened, certain characteristics would dominate all aspects of its growth and perinatal development into toddlerhood.

The enslaved African had become preferred for servitude over the indentured servant in spite of the front-end investment that exceeded costs associated with utilizing indentured servants. As a result, the demand for enslaved Africans to support the remuneration of investments back to English financiers increased exponentially. In addition, the cost of enslaved Africans being brought to the "New World" from malarial nations was higher than those from less impacted areas on the continent. These two factors demonstrate colonial ability to facilitate the development of a merchant market that used markers of bio-geographic specificity to select the "chattel" that would provide the highest production yield. This was one of many castigations aimed at the sub-Saharan African for bio-ecological predispositions over which they had no control; others include skin color, religion of birth, language and region of origin (Esposito, 2015).

In Conclusion

The importance in identifying how individuals, organizations and groups gain the motivation to engage in the behaviors and activities in which they do cannot be over-stated. The institution of slavery is often analyzed absent a detailed analysis of how and why it came to be. Many scholars discuss the slave trade in isolation, disconnected from the contexts in which it was born. History provides an array of patterns and pre-texts that when studied are often predictable and preventable.

Our current world continues to witness racism, misogyny, homophobia, xenophobia, classism and a host of other hateful and hurtful paradigms. Whether we assess legislation, the development of organizations and institutions, warfare or economics, it is critical to conduct analyses on the associated root causes to these concerns and conditions.

Understanding the "why" is just one portion to this intricately and deliberately woven quilt of conquest and destruction. What tools were used to grow and maintain these oppressive systems? How did the key players get involved? Why did the system grow and thrive? Once one understands the constructs underlying a predilection to act heinously, they might then be compelled to understand more about how the behaviors manifest themselves across time. The following chapters answer these questions and many more.

REFERENCES

Abramovitz, M., & Albrecht, J. (2013). The Community Los Index: A New Social Indicator. *Social Science Review, 87*(4), 677–723.

Adiele, P. O. (2017). *The Popes, the Catholic Church and the Transatlantic Enslavement of Black Africans 1418–1839.* Hildesheim: Georg Olms Publishing.

Baptiste, E. (2015). *The Half Has Never Been Told: Slavery and the Making of Modern Capitalism.* New York: Basic Books.

Berquist Soule, E. (2017). From Africa to the Ocean Sea: Atlantic Slavery in the Origins of the Spanish Empire. *Atlantic Studies, 15*(1), 16–39.

Bonikowski, B. (2016). Nationalism in Settled Times. *The Annual Review of Sociology, 2016*(42), 427–449. Harvard University.

Davenport, F. G. (2004). *European Treaties Bearing on the History of the United States and Its Dependencies to 1648.* Clark, NJ: The Lawbrook Exchange, LTD.

Davidson, E. (1997). *The Making of Adolf Hitler: The Birth and Rise of Nazism.* Columbia, MO: University of Missouri Press.

Esposito, E. (2015). *Side Effects of Immunities: The African Slave Trade.* Florence: European University Institute, Max Weber Programme.

Green, D. (2014). *The Hundred Years War: A People's History.* New Haven, CT: Yale University Press.

Hamilton, R., & Herwig, H. (Eds.). (2003). *The Origins of World War I.* Cambridge: Cambridge University Press.

Hass, E. B. (1986). What Is Nationalism and Why Should We Study It? *International Organization, 40*(3), 707–744. MIT Press.

Jensen, L. (Ed.). (2016). *The Roots of Nationalism: National Identity Formation in Early Modern Europe, 1600–1815* (Heritage and Memory Studies). Amsterdam: Amsterdam University Press.

Kelsey, H. (2003). *Sir John Hawkins: Queen Elizabeth's Slave Trader.* New Haven, CT: Yale University Press.

Mallard, R. Q. (1892). *Plantation Life Before Emancipation.* Richmond, VA: Wittet & Shepperson.

Mann, C. (2014). *1493 for Young People: From Columbus's Voyage to Globalization (For Young People Series).* New York: Seven Stories Press.

Neiberg, M. (2017). *The Treaty of Versailles: A Concise History*. New York: Oxford University Press.

Quijano, A., & Ennis, M. (2000). Coloniality of Power, Eurocentrism and Latin America. *Nepantla: Views from South, 1*(3), 533–580. Duke University Press.

Rivers, C. (Ed.). (2015). *The Rise of Nazi Germany: The History of Events That Brought Adolf Hitler to Power*. Charles Rivers Editors.

Rooney, J., & Vanden-Heuvel, L. (2004, July). Root Cause Analysis for Beginners. *Quality Progress*, 45–53. Retrieved July 8, 2018, from https://www.env.nm.gov/aqb/Proposed_Regs/Part_7_Excess_Emissions/NMED_Exhibit_18-Root_Cause_Analysis_for_Beginners.pdf

Santana, J., Fregel, R., Lightfoot, E., Morales, J., Alamon, M., Guillen, J., et al. (2016). The Early Colonial Atlantic World: New Insights on the African Diaspora from Isotopic and Ancient DNA Analyses of a Multiethnic 15th-17th Century Burial Population from the Canary Islands, Spain. *American Journal of Physical Anthropology, 159*(2), 300–312.

Smith, A. (1994). *The Wealth of Nations*. New York: The Modern Library.

Taylor, E. (2015). *The Fall of the Dynasties: The Collapse of the Old Order: 1905–1922*. New York: Skyhorse Publishing.

Thomas, H. (2014). *The Slave Trade: The Story of the Atlantic Slave Trade: 1440–1870*. New York: Simon & Schuster Paperbacks.

Wallerstein, I. (2004). *World Systems Analysis: An Introduction*. Durham, NC: Duke University Press.

Watson, A. (2014). *Ring of Steel: Germany and Austria-Hungary in World War I, the People's War*. New York: Basic Books.

White, A. (2005). The Changing Adolescent Brain. *Education Canada, 45*(2), 4–6.

Whitfield, C. L., Dube, S., Felitti, V., & Anda, R. (2005). Adverse Childhood Experiences and Hallucinations. *Child Abuse & Neglect, 29*(7), 797–810.

Wilde, R. (2018, May 22). *Aftermath of the Hundred Years War*. Retrieved from https://www.thoughtco.com/aftermath-of-the-hundred-years-war-1221904

CHAPTER 3

Cross-Continental Nooses: *Catalyzed Cotton and Industrial Wealth*

According to the Brookings Institute, Silicon Valley, a collection of municipalities in the southern region of the San Francisco Bay Area of Northern California has the third highest gross domestic product (GDP) per capita in the world. In other words, the combination of capitol, goods and monetized services produced in that region when compared to the population of that same region is higher than most other areas. This status changes with fluctuations in the gross domestic products bred in the region or with population vacillations. As of 2017, over 50 of the world's Fortune 500 companies listed were headquartered in the state of California. More than 20 of these companies sit in Silicon Valley alongside thousands of other start-up enterprises in the region. Companies like Facebook made its first appearance on the list in 2017 at 482, while organizations like Apple, Hewlett Packard, Google, Safeway, Intel and Cisco maintain consistent presence in the top 100 (Metropolitan Policy Program at Brookings, 2018). How is it that this small, obscure geographical space becomes one of the world's most influential economic power players?

In 1899 during the summer before the turn of the century, the very first "ship to shore" wireless telegraph message was received in the USA. A fleet of American ships returning from the Philippines after a victory in the Spanish–American War were able to send a telegraph to shore announcing their return. This area had long been a major hub of United States Naval research and development, renowned institutions of higher learning and the advances in technology and innovation that often accompany these condi-

© The Author(s) 2019
D. E. Grant Jr., *Black Men, Intergenerational Colonialism, and Behavioral Health*, https://doi.org/10.1007/978-3-030-21114-1_3

tions. The first American radio station with regularly scheduled programming was started by Charles Herrold in the region in 1909. Simultaneous to this were the technological developments leading up to the Federal Telegraph Corporation's (FTC) decade long work to establish the world's first global radio communication system. The FTC would gain a contract with the US Navy who would eventually commission a Naval Air Station in the Bay Area, followed by some of the area's first technology firms to support the quickly growing research and development (Cohen, 2017; Metropolitan Policy Program at Brookings, 2018; Wessner, 2013).

Across this time, regions throughout the American west were just developing their sense of American nationalism. Much of the land had recently been annexed and, unlike the eastern seaboard, had not yet experienced the long history of intracontinental cooperative engagement that created a sense of American regional pride, like that of the American Confederacy decades before. Many leaders in the growing western region felt a need to build regional economies that could reduce the paternalistic exploitation they perceived from the east. Frederick Terman, Stanford University's dean of engineering in the 1940s and 1950s, is often referred to as the "Father of the Silicon Valley". He used the university's history of regional engagement with the burgeoning tech industry to build a strong and strategic plan of collaboration and private financial support that would spark the growth of a new economy the world had never before seen. He encouraged collaboration between students, graduates, private companies and the government. In 1951, he proposed that the Stanford Industrial Park lease land to companies dedicated to high technology jobs that their graduates would have access to. He would go on to support these businesses by creating academic partnerships with companies for their employees to pursue graduate degrees and by procuring venture capital for civilian technology start-ups (Cohen, 2017; Metropolitan Policy Program at Brookings, 2018; Wealth X, 2018).

After fear generated by the Russian launch of the world's first space satellite in 1957, the National Aeronautics and Space Act was signed by the President Eisenhower, and its first contract was to Fairchild Semiconductor in the heart of the Silicon Valley. This strategic multi-disciplinary partnership between the federal, private and academic sectors proved fruitful. Silicon Valley would lead the world in technological advancements and the building of an economic and entrepreneurial web that mirrored other historic economic markets. Geographic placement during the Spanish–American War rendered the Silicon Valley an important port for the US Navy. The technology needs of the Navy drew some natural synergies that were recognized by scientists, academics, entrepreneurs and business people. As a result of space and time, innovations grew quickly, catalyzing the regions expertise, productivity and prosperity. In 2017, the Wealth-X 2018 census counted 2754 billionaires across the world. Of these billionaires, 884 live in America, 74 (9%) of that 844 live in the Silicon Valley, placing the region at number three on the list of global regions most inhabited by billionaires (Wealth X, 2018). In addition, these primarily tech billionaires of the Silicon Valley average a higher degree of wealth when compared to non-tech billionaires. It is safe to say that the deliberate and strategic efforts to capitalize on the region's talents and assets have been effective over the past decades to convert this historic farming region to tech giant of the world.

To promote opportunities for analyses with an exhaustively critical lens, it is incumbent upon investigators to assess relevant variables as individual parts of a larger and more complex inter-dependent whole. Researchers and scholars too often aggregate factors that should be explored individually but not independently. Deciding (actively or passively) to ignore details of unique contributions individual variables make to the whole often results in sub-critical and superficial analyses of the condition(s) in question. The orchards across the "Valley of the Hearts Delight", as the region was historically known, would soon be replaced by technology companies, and the region would be rebranded as Silicon Valley in the early 1970s. Contributions from the Navy, Russia's Sputnik launch, Stanford University and engineers across the region can be traced to the creation of a successful and sustained high technology industry that changed the entire world (Cohen, 2017; Metropolitan Policy Program at Brookings, 2018; Wealth X, 2018). Bodies of knowledge that feature this process of detailed change analysis are often welcomed when the identified rubric of success maintains congruence between ethical and moral foundations. Analyses of the "successes" of an industry or institution built upon an amoral foundation create, for many, a level of unpalatable and untenable cognitive dissonance. With the goal of dismantling the mysticism associated with the development of one of the world's biggest tragedies, a detailed exploration in the etiology of the successfully devastating institution of American slavery is required.

When the institution of slavery is explored absent analyses of individual variables that synergized into the whole, we lose the true portrait of intricacies interlocking many of the key players (people, countries religions, industries) in this global massacre. Monsignor Theophilus Okere, Nigerian philosopher and researcher, describes the Transatlantic Slave Trade and the institution of enslavement as "Four Hundred years of European, Christian cruelty, of papally and theologically sanctioned inhumanity that afflicted on Africa a loss in men, in happiness, freedom and dignity" (Adiele, 2017, p. 3). Although we have thoroughly explored the colonial and imperialistic actions of implicated stakeholders, these factors are separate from but not independent of the actual imperialistic practices that sustained the institution of enslavement.

CORPORATE CONGLOMERATES OF ENSLAVEMENT

Estimates indicate that from the time of their entry into the trade of Africans through 1807, when they abolished the practice, the British captured and transported over 3 million enslaved Africans on their ships. They would forcibly introduce 2.7 million of these souls to colonies and countries around the world (Milner, 1890). The first African people to be sold into slavery by the British were pirated from a Portuguese ship by Sir John Hawkins in the mid-sixteenth century. Although late in gaining entry into the industry of African enslavement and the transport of these individuals for other nations, England would soon be the most formidable force of the entire trade, its longevity and its global economic impact across more than four centuries (Kelsey, 2003).

Sir John Hawkins was born in Plymouth, UK, to a prominent family over 130 years after Prince Henry the Navigator of Portugal. He would become one of Great Britain's most renowned maritime explorers, educators and navigators. His dad found success in the mercantile markets, on the seas and in the English Parliament as a principal sea captain for Henry VIII. Exploring the synergistic effects of time and space on an individuals' development of expertise in a specific area or profession plays a significant role in understanding the entire system. As a result of this specific time and space into which John Hawkins was born, he was able to master a unique set of combined skills shortly after his predecessors had made great maritime advances all while his father provided him with access to and experience in essential seafaring skills and strategies. This all occurred in a space where the spoils of imperialism were economically life changing atop a geography perfectly situated to capitalize on these combined factors (Encyclopedia Britannica; Kelsey, 2003).

In 1553, a group of merchant mariners traveled from England to the Guinea Coast where the Portuguese had benefitted from Catholic Church ordained trade monopolies (Ascientos) for over a century. As a result, these 1st English traders were essentially sixteenth-century pirates in violation of the treaties in place that had rendered the Spanish and Portuguese the biggest stakeholders in the enslavement of Black Africans of the time. The first English traders returned to London with pepper, ivory, gold and five African men from Shama, a small Ghanaian fishing town at the mouth of the Pra River. They learned English and were made to serve as intermediaries for traders. Within five years, they were all returned home safely. Sir John Hawkins would lead an expedition seven years later, in 1562, where he would capture a Portuguese ship filled with Africans en-route to their new fate. Hawkins would sell the 300 captives he pirated to sugar planters in the Dominican Republic, making himself a huge profit. His subsequent voyages would be specifically aimed at capturing and selling Africans into perpetual enslavement for profit. Hawkins pioneered the English slave trade by demonstrating that its wealth potential was even greater than that of the gold trade, one of the reasons Britain originally led expeditions into Africa (Kelsey, 2003; Livingstone Smith, 2011).

At this time the English holdings in North America were farming tobacco to export to Europe where it was in high demand. English businessmen made large investments in the success of the British colonies, and they expected the lucrative returns they were promised. The only way to catalyze an economy in a developing nation is to extract natural resources (oil, gold, diamonds, etc.) or cultivate and harvest a crop that holds value on the international market. There were no known precious metals in North America at this time, particularly in the Atlantic colonies. In order to maximize profitability, colonists aimed to increase their tobacco yields. Due to the limits associated with most all crop farming, the most viable way to increase harvests year over year was to increase the actual area of land on which the crop could be grown. Although there was no shortage of land where tobacco could be farmed in the colonies, there was a shortage of land instantaneously ready to welcome the cultivation of this cash crop (Gordon, 2017; Kulikoff, 1986; Thomas, 2014).

The English colonies initially relied upon indentured servants for the labor necessary to cultivate land for crops. Many of them were Europeans working off the terms of their criminal sentence or the cost of their travel to the new land of promise. Even with the temporary European workers, there was still a need for more labor, particularly labor that could sustain life in the newly disease-ridden southern colonies. Due to the shortage of laborers in England, domestic wages were too high to entice more English indentured servants to the colonies. Although there were plenty of poor people looking for work in Scotland and Wales, they, like the other residents of Great Britain, died in great numbers to malaria and yellow fever. The colonists' final decision soon became clear. Europeans were three to five times more likely to die in their first year in the colonies compared to Africans (Esposito, 2015; Mann, 2014). In order to effectively build the nation, a huge escalation in the capture and importation of African people for the purpose of perpetual servitude had to be established. Between 1680 and 1700, the enslaved African population in Virginia grew by over 500%, while the numbers of indentured servants dropped exponentially. Equally as striking as the rate of growth are the specific regions of the continent where the enslaved would be captured (Baptiste, 2015; Robins, 2012).

The Company of Royal Adventurers Trading in Africa was an English trading conglomerate chartered by the House of Stuart and local merchants of London in 1660 to capitalize on West African gold. Its list of investors included Charles II, John Locke, Edmund Andros and Prince Rupert. The English Crown provided them with an Asciento resulting in a complete monopoly over English trade along Africa's western coast. As a part of the agreement, England was tasked with delivering enslaved people to the colonies, supplying the Spanish crown a hearty advance and providing a portion of the profit of the trade directly to the kings of England and Spain. This monopoly was operationalized by the support and protection of both the Royal Army and Navy whose practice of intercepting ships of independent English traders not affiliated with the company and seizing their cargo was critical to the monopoly. This would also mark a sharp rise in the numbers of slave ships arriving to the African coast (Newsweek, 2003; Robins, 2012).

Bunce Island became England's first slave fortress, established in the seventeenth century and situated in the middle of an estuary in the Sierra Leone River. Estuaries are bodies of water that usually mark the intermingling of ocean and intra-continental waters. Various estuaries would serve as points of disembarkment for millions of enslaved African people delivered to foreign lands around the world. This particular estuary was perfect for the ocean faring vessels of that time, leading the British to erect its slave castle there. Millions of enslaved Africans were brought, sold and imprisoned on this island prior to departure (Quinn, 2000; Walvin, 2011).

In 1664, James Duke of York, the future King James II, was the Royal Navy Admiral responsible for the annexation of New Amsterdam, a Dutch colony in the Americas. He would repurpose warehouses and port structures formerly governed by the Dutch West Indian Company, to support his efforts as primary shareholder in the Company of Royal Adventurers Trading in Africa. New Amsterdam would later be renamed New York in his honor. In 1672, the Duke of York would lead a corporate merger between the trading company and the Gambia Merchant's Company to form the Royal African Company (RAC), for which he served as Governor, the modern equivalent to the highest C-Suite executive. Under his leadership, the RAC would be responsible for the transport thousands of enslaved Africans, most of whom had the initials "RAC" or "DY" for Duke of York burned into their flesh as brands, providing both literal and figurative scars as they began their new lives, on this new land, in their new role as "slave" (Newsweek, 2003; Pettigrew, 2016).

Between 1680 and 1688, the RAC deployed 249 ships to the African coast where they captured 60,783 people to enslave. After losing almost 25% of them across the trans-Atlantic trade route, they would deliver 46,396 Africans to the Americas to live out the remainder of their days in bondage (Huggins & Jackson, 2015). By the eighteenth century, independent merchants in England saw the growth in this burgeoning industry and fought for their right to be slave traders using the English constitution as justification. They would effectively break the monopoly created by the Ascientos partially resulting in the exponential growth of the trading of people from the coasts and interiors of the African continent. This open market resulted in year over year increases in the population of enslaved Africans, and their African American children on the plantations of the continental and island colonies of America (Newsweek, 2003; Pettigrew, 2016).

Research demonstrates that besides mercantile greed, there were several factors that contributed to the ecological growth of colonial slavery. The first wave throughout the seventeenth and eighteenth centuries was fueled by both the Native American genocide and the cultivation of tobacco and sugar cane. The second was as a result of the cultivation of cotton and the British Industrial Revolution (Kulikoff, 1986; Robins, 2012).

WHITE GOLD

The British East India Company was established in 1600 to get a hand in the long-time trade between Asia and Europe that Portugal had participated in across the fifteenth century. Followed by the Netherlands and Denmark, these trading companies employed war-like tactics to gain more and more control of the international oceanic trade of silk, cotton and other textiles. Each of these European companies relied upon India for cotton production with which they built the foundations of an international system of trade that would eventually span four continents. The English textile industry throughout the fifteenth and sixteenth centuries had been dominated by the artistry of Asia and the Middle East (Quinn, 2000; Robins, 2012).

The cotton plant is thought to have grown on Earth for over 10 million years across a band of global geography that hosts temperatures remaining above 50 °F with no frost for two-thirds of the year and rains that accumulate to over 20 inches annually (Beckert, 2014). This particular region would include a corridor of modern-day countries and regions from west to east like Mexico, the Southern United States, Peru, Hispaniola, Senegal, Cote d'Ivoire, Sicily, Egypt, Nubia, Anatolia, Persia, Gujarat, Bengal and Southern China. Indigenous people in these lands have been growing and cultivating cotton for centuries. Both independently and interdependently, the first weavers of these nations developed methods that took raw cotton and converted it to colorful cloths, fabrics and textiles (Beckert, 2014).

Interestingly enough, Europe rarely appears in the world's long history of cotton use, cultivation or manufacturing prior to the twelfth century. Europe depended primarily upon wool for all textiles. They had been using wool, flax (linen) and hemp through the seventeenth century when silk was introduced by French religious refugees. Cotton was an exotic plant to Europe, so much so that in 1887 "The Vegetable Lamb of Tartary" by Henry Lee was published to chronicle the long-held belief across Medieval Europe that cotton was actually a hybrid plant-animal that grew from the ground and bore fruit. That fruit was thought to be an actual living lamb attached to the ground. Other reports from traders and explorers describe a lamb suspended above ground by a flexible stalk attached to its naval that allowed it to bend and graze (Lee, 1887). Debates across centuries between scientist and other learned men detail the fantastical explanations they provided for a plant that had been likely cultivated since the beginning of Earth's human inhabitance (Beckert, 2014; Lee, 1887).

Archaeological records demonstrate that the oldest documented practices of spinning and weaving cotton were found in modern-day Pakistan and dated between 3250 and 2750 BCE. For millennia, India was the world's leader in the cultivation and manufacturing of cotton. They weren't alone, however. Cotton fishing nets found in Peru have been dated back to 2400 BCE, and cotton threads from Mexico have been dated back to 1200 BCE. It is even believed that the Nubians were cultivating cotton as early as 5000 BCE. In the Pre-Columbian period, Native Americans and indigenous people across the Caribbean relied upon the cultivation and production of cotton. England wouldn't widely adopt the practice of using cotton for textiles until the seventeenth century (Beckert, 2014; Wessner, 2013).

Wool production was a sacred practice in England and governed by very specific guidelines that effectively limited the quantity of wool that could be produced in any given space of time. Silk, although luxurious and sought after, was expensive and very delicate to work with. As a result, toward the end of the seventeenth century, the East India Company began exporting cotton to England. Compared to wool and silk, cotton was cheap, durable and not subject to production restrictions. Fustian—a linen cotton blend—was introduced to London and eventually overtook its predecessor, the woolen industry. Early in seventeenth century Europe, processes for dying cotton and cotton blends were inefficient at best. The colors didn't take well to the fabric, and the integrity of the color was consistently compromised after washing. The process of calico printing arrived in London in 1675 and effectively imitated the colorful textiles that had been arriving from Asia through the East India Company. Once the English learned to create certain patterns and dying techniques, they became perfectly positioned to dominate this trade, and reliance upon the importation of textiles became less and less important (Beckert, 2014; Quijano & Ennis, 2000; Wessner, 2013).

English merchants were now able to create and sell their colorful textiles at half the cost of the imports. The Indian artisans were not pleased with this new innovation and compelled Parliament to prohibit the sale and use of the plagiarized English calicoes. As a result, the creation of certain patterned fabrics was banned in the UK. The Parliamentary ruling did, however, allow the English artisans to print on fustians which became almost indistinguishable from the calicoes. This presented a huge opportunity for the small northwest English village of Lancashire to serve as the centralized geographic location for the start of the European

Industrial Revolution and global capitalism (Beckert, 2014; Quijano & Ennis, 2000; Wessner, 2013).

The Industrial Revolution began in England in the mid-eighteenth century. It would last for over 50 years, driven by commerce connected to coal mining, hydro and steam power, chemical engineering, and iron making. Although innovation and/or mechanization in each of those arenas stimulated the British economy, it was the textile industry that generated the largest domestic and global impact. Since most goods sourced from raw materials were processed in peoples' homes, the time prior to the Industrial Revolution is often referred to as the "Cottage Industry". The inefficiencies associated with this structure limited production due to restricted capacity. This capacity would soon change with the invention and refinement of several important machines and workshops, both markers of industrialization (Beckert, 2014; Chapmann, 1972).

Italy had been importing cotton from the Mediterranean since the eleventh century, sending threads and raw materials to the homes of skilled weavers who had developed an expertise in the wool industry. By the twelfth century, they had adopted advanced methods of weaving from India and China by proxy of Islamic influence and proximity, making them Europe's first cotton hub. The "Liverpool of the twelfth century", Venice at that time was a bustling port with traders whose sole work was the cotton trade (Beckert, 2014). Germany, who sourced raw cotton from the same Mediterranean lands as the Italians, would soon interrupt their monopoly. They identified less expensive laborers in the German countryside to manufacture textiles and used this cost savings to acquire Italian export markets. Both industries would grow for several generations and both would soon fail. Their access to cotton was restricted. Organized weavers and guild restrictions inflated production costs in Italy, and each country's geography and climate had no capacity to support domestic cultivation. The final straw to effectively halt the mass success of the Northern Italian and Southern German cotton industries was the rise of the Ottoman Empire and their control of trade routes across the Mediterranean. To increase focus on the cultivation of domestic industries, the Ottoman Empire restricted the export of cotton. Without recourse or control, Italy and Germany had no choice but to succumb to the producers' restrictions. It appears that the architects of Britain's approach to cotton production took cues from errors of their European neighbors; strict control of the raw material and those who produce it was key to the growth and sustainability in this age old industry (Baptiste, 2015; Beckert, 2014; Wessner, 2013).

The earliest mention of cotton in English history is in 1601, and in less than two decades British cotton manufacturers were exporting textiles across Europe. Although Lancashire was a major hub of the English Cottage Industry, its growth was slow due to the restrictions present absent workshops that could grow to the mass production capacity of factories. It took almost 80 years, from 1687, for the amount of raw cotton manufacturing to double from 1.9 million pounds to 3.8 million pounds. By 1858, America alone would export this quantity in one day. Even with the slow growth in Lancashire's early days, the weavers who were experts in wool working quickly began to develop technology alongside counterparts in London to mechanize their processes (Baptiste, 2015; Beckert, 2014).

Across three centuries, Europe and North America had been mastering their international partnerships. Britain would serve the partnership in the role of both raw goods consumer and products manufacturer, while America served as both producer and labor driver. Cotton textiles, furnishings and clothing were Britain's biggest export during the time of American slavery. Tobacco had been America's number one plantation economy crop exported to Europe since the inception of the African slave trade; this would soon change. After the arrival of the first small American cotton import to England in 1785, interest in American cotton cultivation grew from notion to necessity (Beckert, 2014; Wessner, 2013).

Cotton was indigenous to the Southern states of America and had been grown for local and personal use long before the first settlers arrived in Jamestown, Virginia. Government officials from James Madison to George Washington vehemently rallied national support for the development of a cotton industry in the American south. There were several factors that contributed to the extreme growth of the American cotton industry and its ascendance to the number one spot of American exports. Through skilled contributions from the Haitian revolution of 1791, the emergent labor market in northwest Britain and innovations in tools and processes on both sides of the Atlantic and American land expansion, their desires for cotton's future would soon be realized (Beckert, 2014; Wessner, 2013).

Haiti and American Cotton

France's first successful colony, Saint-Domingue, which is Haiti today, was founded in the Caribbean in the late 1600s. Sixteenth-century French buccaneers were pirates who lived on small Caribbean islands off the coast of Saint-Domingue and made their living robbing Spanish ships. By the seventeenth century, many of the buccaneers had turned in their tricorns for plantation hats in the new colony. By the 1780s, over half of all of France's foreign investments were based on Saint-Domingue's economy. The colony amassed great wealth as a result of their sugar, coffee, cacao and cotton production. By the eighteenth century, Saint-Domingue was one of the wealthiest European colonies. The French transported over a million enslaved Africans across the Atlantic Ocean to these new colonies during their participation in the trade (Baptiste, 2015; Fleming, 2011; Wessner, 2013).

The Revolution of Haiti began in 1791 and would last for over a decade, ending with the dissolution of the French colony in 1804. Françoise Mackandal, enslaved as a child, was the leader of the Haitian Maroon communities—escaped slaves and natives of a land's interior—in Saint-Domingue. Mackandal was known for making poisons from herbs he found on the island. He sent terror across the island as thousands of colonists were poisoned to death. Enslaved people would secretly add Mackandal's poisons to the meals they served their White enslavers. They even poisoned other enslaved Blacks who they couldn't trust to join their fight for freedom (Geggus, 2014; Girard, 2016).

The French were sure that Mackandal was going to be the death of their colony and the wealth it produced. In addition to his mass poisonings, he led raids on plantations and helped to free many enslaved Haitians. The French eventually found one of Mackandal's allies, an enslaved woman who they tortured to gain information on how to capture him. When the French finally found him, they tortured him and burned him alive in the towns square. Most of the plantation owners brought all the people they owned to the square to witness his torture and burning. They wanted to scare them from even thinking of revolting, as this was a common tool used by enslavers across the world. Some were scared by this demonstration, and many others were emboldened in their fight against enslavement and used Mackandal as inspiration to fuel their work.

Mackandal's efforts preceded Toussaint l'Ouverture's and laid the ground for the final liberation of the island. L'Ouverture's rebellion created a significant gap in the raw material market for European textile producers. Although America was preparing to fill that fissure, the most noteworthy contribution of the Haitian Revolution on the American cotton industry was not the void in supply it created, but the skills of French immigrants and their fear of an empowered enslaved population. The immigration of French planters from Saint-Domingue to different parts of the American south provided an expertise in cotton cultivation that was lacking in the American south. These planters had been complicit in the financial success of the Caribbean colony that brought such great wealth to France and would bring those tools to America as they fled the fate of many White French colonists on the island (Geggus, 2014; Girard, 2016).

The liberation of Haiti was the first successful revolt of free and enslaved Blacks. This had a profound impact on the psyche of the American planter. Fear and terror regarding how the news of this revolution might impact the enslaved Blacks in North America was untenable for the American planter. The panic created by this revolt generated a level of terror in the American planters that impacted their plantation management approaches. In 1791, the year the Haitian Liberation began, American annual cotton production was slightly below 2 million pounds; in just one decade this same land was producing almost 50 million pounds of cotton annually (Beckert, 2014; Geggus, 2014; Girard, 2016).

Hundreds of thousands of people were employed in the cotton mills and factories in Britain. Demographic data from the time indicate that for each mill worker there were at least three other professions supported (tailors, seamstresses, artisans, etc.), demonstrating that most all people in England were reliant upon cotton in some capacity. As an ideal location for the processing of cotton, Lancashire, its surrounding towns and parish all served as the center of the global cotton industry. Synergies between the local climate's ability to sustain strong intact cotton fibers, the hydro-energy powering the mills and the peoples' development of an entrepreneurial empire rendered these Europeans prepared when the opportunity presented itself; it was their time. Most of the families in this region had a member who worked in the mills or in jobs that supported or were supported by the cotton industry. Mid-eighteenth-century baptismal records of Manchester show that 50–70% of fathers identified worked in some domain of the textile industry. In Saddleworth, 11 miles northeast of current Manchester, 85% of the fathers worked in this industry (Baptiste, 2015; Beckert, 2014). These statistics were similar across the entire northwest portion of England and other surrounding areas. Although slave cotton changed the life of the British family across generations, economic historians consistently demonstrate that a reliance of an entire region on one industry always results in extreme consequences, sometimes good, but usually not.

American Innovation and Expansion

In 1792, a young Yale graduate moved to Georgia to rent a room on the plantation of Catherine Greene. In 1780, Greene's husband, Nathanael Greene, was named commander of the Continental Army in the southern theater by George Washington. He would die from heat stroke in 1786 leaving his young wife to manage their struggling plantation and raise their children. By 1793, Catherine had familiarized Eli Whitney—the young graduate—with the toils of cotton cultivation and together they introduced the cotton gin to the American Southern plantation system. When Eli Whitney moved to Catherine Greene's Georgia plantation, she was struggling to make a profit from her cotton crops; that would change with this innovation.

The cotton gin is a machine that facilitates easier cleaning and processing of cotton as it mechanized the separation of the seeds from the fibers that were historically only removed by hand. As a result of this substantial efficiency, plantations were able and expected to harvest more and more cotton each season. This new quantitative expectation could only be met with additional labor as America grew to supply 80% of the world with the cotton they needed to produce their respective goods. In 1800, less than a decade after Greene and Whitney's cotton gin and Samuel Crompton's spinning mule, the consumption of cotton by England increased by 140% to 52 million pounds from 1787 (after textile processing mechanization but before the cotton gin in 1793). From 1800 to 1850, the consumption of cotton in England would grow by over 1000% to close to 600 million pounds. During this same general time period, some notable population shifts also occurred. The population of England grew by over 300% across the entirety of the nineteenth century. Urbanization had begun, and for the first time in English history, there seemed to be a sustainable, reliable and predictable improvement in overall quality of life, health and wellness for the people living within its European continental crown (Beckert, 2014).

Another major contributor to the growth of the cotton industry in America was its land expansion. Three major acquisitions would ensure the prosperity of the American cotton economy. The Louisiana Purchase of 1803 doubled the land mass of the USA of the time. The USA would annex Florida from Spain in 1819 and Texas in 1845. Cotton is a crop that fatigues soil after consistent replanting without the rotation of a different crop. Yields decrease significantly when rotation doesn't occur. The seemingly unlimited land of America allowed new plantations to pop up on fertile parcels as fresh acreage. The land was annexed and its native inhabitants were either forced to cede their land, pushed further west or murdered. By the middle of the nineteenth century, almost 70% of America's cotton was being grown on land that had only been newly acquired since the start of the century (Baptiste, 2015).

America would see a similar socio-economic and quality of life trend among colonizing Whites as did the English with their textile workers. Each of these aforementioned conditions promoting extreme growth could only be possible given an equally extreme increase in the labor force responsible for the production of the crop. At the end of the eighteenth century when the cotton gin was invented, there were fewer than 700,000 enslaved Blacks in America, and just 60 years later there were over 3 million, a more than 300% increase, strikingly congruent with that of Whites in England (Thomas, 2014). Unfortunately, the analogous population explosion would render individuals and families of African descent with a severe decline in quality and longevity of life. Evidence shows that there were many English families disenfranchised during the Industrial Revolution; poverty didn't disappear nor was the entirety of the country riding the wave of prosperity. Having said that, the experience of virtually 100% of all enslaved Blacks in the Americas devolved into a nightmare many thought could not get worse than it had already been. England's thirst for cotton and the brutality of American slavery grew in strength across a pattern of concurrent reciprocity.

Exponential growth is defined as a growth rate that increases in accordance to the growing total of the population. In 1714, the total population of enslaved Blacks in America was 59,000. By 1727, this population had risen to 78,000 and is recorded at 293,000 in 1754, a 275% increase in less than three decades. During the 1760s, it is estimated that 40,000 enslaved people were transported to the colonies in British ships each year resulting in a US Census report showing 697,897 "slaves" in 1790, a 138% increase across just three and a half decades. Fifty years later in 1840, the US Census reported a total of 2,487,355 enslaved Blacks being held as property in the USA, a 256% increase (Huggins & Jackson, 2015; Thomas, 2014).

Exponential growth is a phenomenon that occurs under very specific circumstances. In order for the base of a population or group to grow continuously in direct proportion to itself, certain ecological factors must be in place. Under the right conditions, rabbits will reproduce, algae will divide and atomic nuclei will split at exponential rates. Each of these usu-

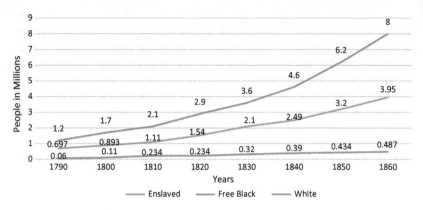

Fig. 3.1   US population 1790–1860

ally result in some disaster, namely: massive crop damage from invasive species infestations, oceanic strangulation and death of sea life from Red Tide algal blooms and atomic bombs which need neither explanation nor additional context.

Figure 3.1 uses US census data to show the population growth between 1790 and 1860, the approximate time between the Haitian Liberation and the abolition of American enslavement (Huggins & Jackson, 2015; Thomas, 2014; US Census).

In the mid-nineteenth century, just prior to the abolition of slavery, parts of the American South and the English Northwest were some of the richest places in the world. Cotton was sent from the American south to processing plants, mills and factories across the globe, but primarily to Britain. The Manchester Chamber of Commerce, one of the world's most industrialized cities of the time, was troubled by the prospects of the future supply of cotton coming from America. They were all thriving business owners in the center of the cotton empire. They had capitalized upon the plantation economy for their cotton supply across centuries. The cotton supply they processed into tapestries, upholstery and clothing for aristocrats, proletariats and enslaved people was now under threat. Lobbying for increased cotton from India, the Chamber along with others like the East India Company and the Bombay Chamber of Commerce enlisted robust efforts to retain their supply, the foundation of their economy at the time (Beckert, 2014).

The countryside, where most of the European population lived prior to nineteenth-century urbanization, had created an experienced workforce and foundation for capitalism long before the Industrial Revolution as merchants from London and other English towns utilized their services for processing raw materials. Sixteenth-century England was home to two-thirds of the world's looms. Raw cotton was processed using 1500 Dutch engine looms housed in workshops across the country, marking one of the first evolutionary steps to the modern-day industrial factory. At the start of the eighteenth century, they were mostly only tasked with weaving fustian cloth to send to London for dying and printing. It wasn't long before they were creating their own colorful textiles and selling them to markets in France and across Europe. These colorful fabrics were also lauded by African traders (Beckert, 2014; Chapmann, 1972).

By the seventeenth and eighteenth centuries, men, women and children—child labor exploitation was prevalent—of England were entrepreneurs and laborers in factories producing and exporting colorful fustians to consumers across the globe. During this same time, White men, women and children—children of planters were often trained to discipline the enslaved—in America mastered tenets of the plantation economy, including but not limited to the use of punitive practices and specific tools of oppression that forced enslaved Blacks to work harder at a faster rate across more hours under the most extreme psychological torment. In 1750, more than 2 million pounds of raw cotton was imported into Britain, and by 1787 they had imported 22 million pounds. This 1000% increase was made possible by the textile machines invented and refined from the 1730s through the 1780s. Patent records for British inventors document weaving machines and spooling advancements that contemporary societies take for granted. Machines like the flying shuttle and the spinning frame, the spinning jenny and the spinning mule all made the process of transforming clean raw cotton into usable fabric exponentially faster, more efficient and less expensive. Entrepreneurs and factories began to pop up simultaneously all around England to support the cotton industry and the others associated with the revolution (Beckert, 2014).

In 1784, entrepreneur Samuel Greg opened and staffed the Quarry Bank Mill on the banks of the Bollin River outside of modern-day Manchester. Greg used a waterfall to power his machines, and for the first time ever, machines converted cotton to thread using hydropower, the weight of falling water. Greg was connected to several aspects of this industry as were many English entrepreneurs. Much of his wealth origi-

nated from the hundreds of enslaved Africans he owned on a sugar plantation in Dominica, not to be confused with the Dominican Republic. In
fact, it was quite common for English entrepreneurs to have business partnerships across several of the intertwined businesses during the Industrial
Revolution. Men like Richard Paley of Leeds partnered in cotton mills,
iron work and real estate while Robert Dunmore added partnership in a
wool company to Paley's same set of business ventures. Although individual bankruptcy records of the time demonstrate credit extensions that
created bankruptcy for many individuals, including Paley and Dunmore,
there were also many manufacturers and businesses that were forced out
of business. In 1788, Livesey, Hargrave & Co, leading calico producers,
filed for bankruptcy. This was after a myriad of cotton mills and auxiliary
businesses were sent under (Beckert, 2014).

Capacity and populations had now grown. Between 1700 and 1800,
Liverpool alone grew from 5000 to 78,000 (Beckert, 2014). The English
had effectively increased the output of processed fabrics from raw cotton
using specialized machines they invented and/or refined. Prior to this
time, there was a ceiling on the amount of raw cotton they could process.
Not only was this no longer the case, they had now also built an entire
lifestyle around the cotton industry. Imports from the colonies, Asia and
the Middle East were no longer sufficient. In order to effectively sustain
the lifestyle created around the industry across England, increased importation of raw cotton was an absolute necessity. After hundreds of years of
stagnancy and slow growth, the British cotton industry would, from 1780
to 1800, experience an annual average growth rate of 10.8% per year for
the manufacture of cotton textiles and a 14% year over year increase in the
export of cotton textiles. The industry was growing rapidly. By the end of
the eighteenth century, Britain had built capacity to produce cotton goods
of the same quality as India and for a comparable or even lower price
across its 900 cotton factories (Beckert, 2014; Wessner, 2013). At this
time, cotton in America was not yet being heavily exported. In fact, the
first American cotton imports that arrived to Liverpool harbor in 1785 on
a ship owned by Peel, Yates & Co were so suspicious that they were
impounded by British customs agents. It wouldn't take long for the British
merchants to realize their dependence on cotton from the West Indies,
Brazil, the Ottoman Empire and India was a significant limiting factor to
their growth and development (Beckert, 2014).

In 1860, there were 2650 cotton mills and processing plants in
Lancashire, northwest Britain and the surrounding areas. These plants

provided employment for almost a half million people. They exported 2.7 billion yards of fabric totaling 32 million pounds (Beckert, 2014). Of all the cotton processed in this region, 80% originated from the American south. There were both supporters and detractors of the Confederacy throughout Europe. French and English journalists mongered fear of an unraveling of their society and added to the Confederate propaganda. Ill-fated attempts at sourcing affordable cotton elsewhere catalyzed this agenda across the country.

The American Civil War was waged and a cotton embargo was enacted to push Britain's hand into supporting the Confederacy all while they had saturated the global market with fabrics and yarns they couldn't sell. It wasn't long before hundreds of mills in Britain were forced to close. Thousands of Brits emigrated from their homeland while thousands of others who remained were evicted from their homes. Soup kitchens were set up, relief from the Poor Law Act was distributed and food rations from across the globe were dispersed. Funds like the Mansion House Committee of London (Lancashire and Cheshire Operatives Relief Fund) and the Central Relief Committee of Manchester provided support for those who were left destitute during the Cotton Famine (Baptiste, 2015; Beckert, 2014; Wessner, 2013).

Some planters were able to repurpose themselves but most weren't and unemployment became the status quo. Although many municipalities chose a side, as a nation, Britain remained formally neutral on official record regarding the outcome of the American Civil War. Liverpool was explicitly supportive of the American south, while the mill workers in Rochdale—a town in Manchester—built Cotton Stone Road, a monument demonstrating their support in the global struggle to abolish slavery in spite of the extreme struggles they were experiencing in their homeland. The situation was so serious that in 1863, Abraham Lincoln penned a letter directly to the "Working-men of Manchester". He wrote, in part:

> When I came ... to preside in the Government of the United States, the country was found at the verge of a civil war ... I know and deeply deplore the sufferings which the working-men of Manchester, and in all Europe, are called to endure in this crisis. It has been often and studiously represented that the attempt to overthrow this government, which was built on the foundation of human rights, and to substitute for it one which should rest exclusively on the basis of human slavery, was likely to obtain the favor of Europe. Through the action of our disloyal citizens, the working-men of Europe have been subjected to severe trials, for the purposes of forcing their

sanction to that attempt ... I hail this interchange of sentiment, therefore, as an augury that whatever else may happen, whatever misfortune may befall your country or my own, the peace and friendship which now exists between the two nations will be, as it shall be my desire to make them, perpetual. (Littell, 1863, p. 518)

A monument and town square (Lincoln Square) were dedicated to Lincoln in Manchester in 1919 to acknowledge his personal and legislative support of the English mill workers during the Cotton Famine. As domestic battles on both fronts—north and south—began to brew surrounding the moral ground on which the institution of slavery stood, confederates were bred and unionists were emboldened, further endangering British cotton imports.

The Southern planter had maintained a strong monopoly on cotton production and exportation across the globe. The business they created appeared to be full-proof, and by all accounts, its longevity here to fore had shown a successful business model that was sustainable across generations. As a result of this success, these American politicians, war heroes, slave drivers and business owners were arrogantly confident that any behaviors they exhibited would garner support from the international community, even something as extreme as cessation.

James Henry Hammond, South Carolinian, Senator and 60th governor of South Carolina epitomized the southern planters' mentality. He demonstrated an egocentrism congruent with the wealth and influence that resulted from he and his constituency's participation in an international cotton industry built on the backs of enslaved people. In 1858, while addressing the United States Congress, the then Senator of South Carolina notes the following:

Without firing a gun, without drawing a sword, should they make war on us, we could bring the whole world to our feet. The South is willing to go on one, two, or three years without planting a seed of cotton ... What would happen if no cotton was furnished for three years? ... England would topple headlong and carry the whole civilized world with her save the South. No, you dare not to make war on cotton. No power on earth dares to make war upon it. Cotton is king. (Yafa, 2006)

Hammond would go on to reference reports from the 1857 US Secretary of the Treasury to explain to the other Senators in the room that the American South was responsible for exports and products that far exceeded any output of the Northern states. According to Hammond, 66% of the US-exported domestic yields were

> the clear produce of the South; articles that are not and cannot be made at the North ... the *recorded* exports of the South now are greater than the whole exports of the United States in any year before 1856. They are greater than the whole average exports of the United States for the last 12 years ... there is not a nation on the face of the earth, with any numerous population, that can compete with us in produce *per capita*. (Hammond, 1866, pp. 314–315)

This evidence-informed rhetoric ignited an egotism that fanned the flames of cessation propaganda soon to take hold of the American south. "The Republican party of the United States was born of a negroized fanaticism, and hypo-philanthrophy for the negro now constitutes the active element or moving principles of the party. Eliminate this element from this party and it never would have been formed ... and our civil war would not have started" (Milner, 1890, p. 5). Steps toward secession quickened shortly after the election of Republican President Abraham Lincoln in November 1860. South Carolina was the very first state to secede from the Union in December of 1860. Mississippi would follow less than a month later. Joined by five other southern states, they formed the Confederate States of America in February 1861. Jefferson Davis was their first and only president. After the American Civil War began, other states that continued to enslave Black Americans seceded from the USA and joined the Confederacy (Baptiste, 2015; Metropolitan Policy Program at Brookings, 2018).

Emanuel Lehman—the German-Jewish son of a cattle dealer—immigrated to Alabama in the 1840s after learning about the big cotton boom in the USA. Upon arrival, he began selling goods up and down the Alabama River that he was able to get on credit from a Jewish wholesale merchant familiar with his family back home. Soon after, Emanuel and his brother would have made enough revenue peddling goods that they would be able to open up their own specialty store, Lehman & Bro, right across the road from Montgomery's slave auction block. In 1850, Mayer, a third brother, would arrive and the store would be renamed Lehman Brothers (Cox, 2008; National Archives, 2018).

"The racial inferiority of the colonized implied that they were not worthy of wages. They were naturally obliged to work for the profit of their owners" (Quijano & Ennis, 2000, p. 539). The juxtaposition of the White American and European narrative to the Black African, Caribbean and American narrative of this time period forecasts a sharp difference that would manifest across centuries into modern times. Intergenerational advantage is the accumulation of wealth, power and influence across generations. Many of the businesses that started during the times of enslavement thrived across space and time resulting in and/or facilitating generations of power, affluence and influence.

Lehman Brothers operated largely on a barter system through which they had also become cotton brokers. The farmers would often come to get supplies and exchange them for cotton that the brothers would then turn into cash. This and other businesses like it provided a great foundation for planters to grow their farms. Soon, the brothers began buying land and selling land. This would allow them to extend long range credit to planters. In 1858, Emanuel moved to New York and opened up a Lehman Brothers there. They made money trading in commodities like cotton, coffee and petroleum. The company would soon move from merchant banking to investment banking and end up as one of the most successful firms in American history. For over 75 years, every partner had the last name Lehman. They would partner with fellow Jewish immigrant families like the Goldmans and the Sachs of Goldman & Sachs to acquire great wealth by building businesses like Sears and Roebuck. Although neither of these companies—Lehman Brothers or Sears and Roebuck—hold any viability today, they were once two of the most important businesses in the country that would not have existed had it not been for the business of American slavery (Cox, 2008; National Archives, 2018).

There were no established banks in the cities of England until the mid-seventeenth century. A voyage to procure slave cargo leaving from Liverpool to Africa and then on to the Caribbean could take 18 months. Most of those entering the slave trade didn't have enough capital to sustain such a long and expensive trip. They required loans and credit. Liverpool merchants, purchasing goods from colonial planters, eventually formed Heywood's Bank that would become a part of Barclays. Barclays was founded on slave profits from brothers Alexander and David Barclay who were Quaker slave traders in the West Indies. The Bank of England supported the country's system of commercial credit, established primarily out of need for the support of the lucrative slave trade, the naval protection of the monopolized trade routes and the development of the overseas territories (Walvin, 2011).

It was not uncommon in the nineteenth century for planters and slave owners to have insurance policies on the people they had purchased. Some policies were for those on slave ships in transit to them, and others were for the ones they imprisoned on their labor plantations. In 2000, the insurance giant Aetna apologized for providing insurance policies on enslaved people whereby their owners would be reimbursed for losses after their deaths under certain conditions. Court records from insurance claims and denial appeals demonstrate that these companies granted both life and property insurance to the enslavers who owned the policies. Whether enslaved people were released on their way to their point of disembarkment or murdered a mile away from their plantation, the insurance holders had rights to make claims for their "property loss". In 2002, the city of Chicago passed the Slavery Era Disclosure Ordinance. It mirrored a similar California law that compels insurers who did business in America while the institution of slavery was legal, to report the enslaved people they insured and the holders who owned the policies. Chicago's law requires that all businesses entering into contracts with the city file documentation with the city's purchasing department (Newsweek, 2003; Quinn, 2000). In 2002, a class action lawsuit—aggregated from several individual claims—was filed against a group of corporations who themselves or their predecessors had ties to the Transatlantic Slave Trade and created significant unjust wealth from the labor of enslaved Americans. The lawsuit, dismissed in 2005, named JP Morgan Chase, Aetna, R.J Reynolds Tobacco Co, Union Pacific railroads, Lloyd's of London, Fleet Boston Financial Corp and others in the suit, alleging that each organization benefitted financially from a system that enslaved, tortured, starved and demoralized human beings (Leith, 2002; Magill, 2005).

In January 2005, JP Morgan Chase filed a disclosure statement with the city of Chicago acknowledging that both Citizens Bank and Canal Bank of Louisiana accepted approximately 13,000 enslaved African Americans as loan collateral between 1831 and 1865. Citizens and Canal were both predecessors of the banking giant who admits that as a result of their history of participation in the institution of American slavery, they actually owned 1250 of the enslaved people as a result of the defaulted loans. After the disclosure was forced, JP Morgan Chase made an apology and pledged a $5 million scholarship program over five years for Black Louisiana college students (Magill, 2005; Mann, 2014; Quinn, 2000).

Lloyd's Coffee House was an important meeting place in the hub of London's burgeoning financial district during the seventeenth and eighteenth centuries. Opened by Edward Lloyd in 1686, it was frequented by sailors, slavers, traders and shippers to discuss maritime insurance, shipping and overseas trade. It became a reliable source of shipping and maritime news in the region. Lloyd's of London remains today one of the most respected markets in the industry. Men like Lloyd, or Ambrose Crowley, an English iron merchant who gained great wealth making manacles, collars and ankle irons to prevent Africans from running away or jumping from the slave ship, found great wealth. Each would pass that wealth down to their families. Thomas King—partner in Camden, Calvert and King— owned one in five slave ships that sailed from London. He amassed great wealth to pass down to his children like the Lehman brothers, one of whose son, Herbert Henry Lehman, became the 45th governor of New York and a US Senator (Cox, 2008, National Public Radio (NPR), 2003; Robins, 2012).

These White men and millions of others benefited from the intergenerational accumulation of advantage. Their children gained legacies imbued with a history of fortitude and power. No matter whether they were Englishmen on their mainland, German immigrants who became White Americans by throwing away their ethnicity or French colonial plantation owners, they each were able to provide their children with a world where they not just saw themselves as powerful, but omnipotent as their power was mechanized and monetized in almost every facet of international human life that one could think of. This lens makes it second nature for White boys and men, across their development, to see themselves in positions of power and feel entitled to a seat at the table because they consistently saw their fathers and grandfathers, uncles and brothers (biologic or esoteric) in those seats. The consequences of the opposite scenario have the capacity to create a dangerously debilitated sense of self.

In 2003, researchers found that children form occupational stereotypes on the basis of race and that the racial distributions of workers affect their own judgments and aspirations. Results from the adolescents who participated in the study demonstrate that as early as second grade, Black children aspire to more modest careers than White children. Black children tend to assess their limitations according to their family's current socioeconomic status and have awareness of prejudicial attitudes that might exist in workplaces dominated by other ethnicities. Black children receive messages from dominant culture that mere hard work and diligence lead to economic rewards and occupational success. This information is countered by the images they see of hard working and diligent Black men and women who are consistently relegated to the lowest rungs of the workforce and associated socio-economic ladder. As a result of this data, it becomes clear that Black children are disproportionately likely to misinterpret potentialities of their abilities, impacting the route to self-actualization rendering learned helplessness a very viable existence for many Black children (Bigler, Averhart, & Liben, 2003).

Conclusion

The danger of accumulated advantage is the extreme fear of losing it. In 2019, wealthy, largely White American parents were charged—some indicted and arrested—for utilizing bribes and other illegal measures to create a separate and illegal pathway for their children's entry into elite college and university systems. One couple was accused of paying upwards of $500,000 to get their daughters into one of the many elite universities implicated in the conspiracy. As a result, the United States Department of Education was compelled to investigate what appears to be a $25 million scandal where over 50 people were charged. It appears that university agents were bribed, college testing proctors were compromised, student athletic abilities were fabricated and successful students were paid to cheat on tests for prospective students. Although this activity was illegal, the world has a long history of maintaining a legal restrictiveness on access to elite institutions. The proverbial "back door" of elite higher education has always existed. There are countless numbers of mediocre high school graduates of White affluence who gained entry into the Ivy League shortly after their family made a large donation or erected a small building.

To secure this disparity by constricting social mobility and maintaining a system of structural classism, those who experience accumulated advantage work hard to maintain the mechanisms born inside accumulated disadvantage. Black people are faced with consistent barriers associated with gaining economic empowerment, occupational success or career ascension. Researchers report the existence of a severe social mobility concern in America which results in a perceived attainability of affluence disparity among American citizens (Hirschl & Rank, 2015). Blacks and Whites see the world differently when it comes to their varied levels of agency in the attainment of the "American Dream". This plays out as many White families report beliefs that "the system" works for everyone as is evidenced by their lived experience. This paradigm is juxtaposed to those who believe that the system works, but only consistently for those who are White. The Federal Glass Ceiling Commission indicated in its 1995 report that African American children's judgment of "familiar jobs" was linked to their knowledge of racial segregation on these jobs. Prior to this report, it has been widely believed that African American children and adolescents were unaware of the under-representation of African Americans in high status skilled and managerial positions and their over-representation in low status service positions (Federal Glass Ceiling Commission, 1995).

Outcomes for Black boys and men will never reach optimal levels of success when compared to their White male counterparts if our systems don't address the reality that the world's participation in these horrific events lives on today in both tangible and intangible ways. Not only are there statues and relics strategically positioned around the world that celebrate those complicit in Black captivity and commodification, there are contemporarily thriving industries and organizations that were literally built atop the spilled blood of Black men and women stolen from the only lives they knew. They would now raise their children within a system that enslaved them before they were even conceived. And now, centuries beyond the first African captive's nightmare, twenty-first-century Black families continue to receive scars from a system they never touched but know so well through the successful business continuity model expertly implemented.

References

Adiele, P. O. (2017). *The Popes, the Catholic Church and the Transatlantic Enslavement of Black Africans 1418–1839*. Hildesheim: Georg Olms Publishing.

Baptiste, E. (2015). *The Half Has Never Been Told: Slavery and the Making of Modern Capitalism*. New York: Basic Books.

Beckert, S. (2014). *Empire of Cotton: A Global History*. New York: Alfred A. Knopf.

Bigler, R., Averhart, C., & Liben, L. (2003). Race and the Workforce; Occupational Status, Aspirations, and Stereotyping Among African American Children. *Developmental Psychology, 39*(3), 572–580.

Chapmann, S. D. (1972). *The Cotton Industry in the Industrial Revolution*. London: Macmillan Press.

Cohen, P. (2017). *How Cambridge and Silicon Valley Became Startup Hubs*. Forbes. Retrieved from https://www.forbes.com/sites/petercohan/2017/07/18/how-cambridge-and-silicon-valley-became-startup-hubs/#3fd895f137a7

Cox, D. (2008). *Lehman Bros. Link to Slavery.* Workers World. Retrieved from https://www.workers.org/2008/us/lehman_1030/

Encyclopedia Britannica. *Sir John Hawkins.* Retrieved from https://www.britannica.com/biography/John-Hawkins-English-naval-commander

Esposito, E. (2015). *Side Effects of Immunities: The African Slave Trade.* Fiesole: European University Institute, Max Weber Programme.

Federal Glass Ceiling Commission. (1995, March). *Good for Business: Making Full Use of the Nation's Human Capital: The Environmental Scan.* Washington, DC.

Fleming C. M. (2011). *Imagining French Atlantic Slavery: A Comparison of Mnemonic Entrepreneurs and Antillean Migrants in Metropolitan France.* Doctoral Dissertation, Harvard University, Cambridge, MA.

Geggus, D. (2014). *The Haitian Revolution: A Documentary History.* Indianapolis, IN: Hackett Publishing.

Girard, P. (2016). *Toussaint Louverture: A Revolutionary Life.* New York: Basic Books.

Gordon, D. M. (2017). Slavery and Redemption in the Catholic Missions of the Upper Congo, 1878–1909. *Slavery & Abolition, 38*(3), 577–600.

Hammond, J. H. (1866). *Selections from the Letters and Speeches of the Honorable James H. Hammond of South Carolina.* New York: John F. Trow & CO., Printers.

Hirschl, T., & Rank, M. (2015). The Life Course Dynamics of Affluence. *PLoS One, 10*(1), e0116370.

Huggins, W., & Jackson, J. (2015). *Introduction to African Civilizations.* Cambridge: Ravenio Books.

Kelsey, H. (2003). *Sir John Hawkins: Queen Elizabeth's Slave Trader.* New Haven: Yale University Press.

Kulikoff, A. (1986). *Tobacco and Slaves: Development of the Southern Cultures in the Chesapeake, 1680–1800.* Chapel Hill, NC: University of North Carolina Press.

Lee, H. (1887). *Vegetable Lamb of Tartary, A Curious Fable of the Cotton Plant.* London: Sampson Low, Marston, Searle & Rivington.

Leith, S. (2002). *American Firms Sued Over 'Links to Slavery'.* The Telegraph. Retrieved from https://www.telegraph.co.uk/news/worldnews/northamerica/usa/1388918/American-firms-sued-over-links-to-slavery.html

Littell, E. (1863). *Littell's Living Age.* Boston: Littell, Son and Company.

Livingstone Smith, D. (2011). *Less Than Human: Why We Demean, Enslave, and Exterminate Others.* New York: St. Martin's Press.

Magill, K. (2005). *From J.P. Morgan Chase, an Apology and $5 Million in Slavery Reparations.* The New York Sun. Retrieved from https://www.nysun.com/business/from-jp-morgan-chase-an-apology-and-5-million/8580/

Mann, C. (2014). *1493 From Columbus's Voyage to Globalization for Young People.* New York: Seven Stories Press.

Metropolitan Policy Program at Brookings. (2018). *Global Metro Monitor 2018*. Brookings Institute. Retrieved from https://www.brookings.edu/wp-content/uploads/2018/06/Brookings-Metro_Global-Metro-Monitor-2018.pdf

Milner, J. T. (1890). *White Men of Alabama Stand Together: 1860 & 1890*. Birmingham, AL: McDavid Printing Company.

National Archives. (2018). Retrieved from http://www.nationalarchives.gov.uk/help-with-your-research/research-guides/british-transatlantic-slave-trade-records/

National Public Radio (NPR). (2003). *Lehman Brothers Admits to Past Ties to Slavery*. Interview on Morning Edition by Cheryl Corley. Retrieved from https://www.npr.org/templates/story/story.php?storyId=1543861

Newsweek. (2003). *Slavery: Disclosure Time*. Retrieved from https://www.newsweek.com/slavery-disclosure-time-135209

Pettigrew, W. (2016). *Freedom's Debt: The Royal African Company and the Politics of the Atlantic Slave Trade, 1762–1752*. Chapel Hill, NC: University of North Carolina Press.

Quijano, A., & Ennis, M. (2000). Coloniality of Power, Eurocentrism and Latin America. *Nepantla: Views from South, 1*(3), 533–580. Duke University Press.

Quinn, M. S. (2000). Slavery & Insurance Examining Slave Insurance in a World 150 Years Removed. *Insurance Journal*. Retrieved from https://www.insurancejournal.com/magazines/mag-legalbeat/2000/05/15/21120.htm

Robins, N. (2012). *The Corporation the Changed the World*. London: Pluto Press.

Thomas, H. (2014). *The Slave Trade: The Story of the Atlantic Slave Trade: 1440–1870*. New York: Simon & Schuster Paperbacks.

US Census. https://www.census.gov/history/www/genealogy/decennial_census_records/census_records_2.html

Walvin, J. (2011). *Slavery and the Building of Britain*. BBC. Retrieved from http://www.bbc.co.uk/history/british/abolition/building_britain_gallery_02.shtml

Wealth X. (2018). *The Wealth X Billionaire Census 2018*. Retrieved from https://www.wealthx.com/report/the-wealth-x-billionaire-census-2018/?utm_campaign=billionaire-census-2018&utm_source=press&utm_medium=referral&utm_term=bc-2018-press&utm_source=press&utm_medium=referral

Wessner, C. (Ed.). (2013). *Best Practices in State and Regional Innovation Initiatives; Competing in the 21st century*. Washington, DC: National Research Council and The National Academies Press.

Yafa, S. (2006). *Cotton: The Biography of a Revolutionary Fiber*. London: Penguin Books.

CHAPTER 4

Scientific Nooses: *Epigenetics and Contemporary Injuries*

People immersed in their daily lives rarely have the luxury or inclination to explore the nuanced distances between the realities of their experience paralleled to that of those around them. Attempts at understanding the ways in which information acquired during our daily routines manifests itself in our behaviors, responses to external stimuli and emotional wellness present a complicated effort. Theory can be described as a "series of two or more interrelated constructs … concepts, variables … and propositions, which have been hypothesized with a systematic view of phenomena, for the purpose of explaining and predicting the phenomena" (Udo-Akang, 2012, p. 90). Theoretical alignment helps to ensure that bodies of work are reliable, relevant and informed by evidence. Although this text explores a wide range of disciplines; psychology, social psychology, analytical sociology and cultural anthropology are the primary theoretical frameworks used to evaluate, interpret and explain its contents. Contextualizing these disciplines within this work provides a unique opportunity to look at the conditions of Black men and boys across the diaspora though a strength-based lens supported by evidence and conversant in honoring the various factors that impact their existential experiences and conditions of disproportionality across the lifespan.

Psychology is the study of human behavior, while sociology is the study of social relationships and their manifestation in societies throughout the world. Analytical sociology, a specific branch of the discipline, states that the "values, perceptions, emotions, and modes of reasoning of the actor

© The Author(s) 2019

D. E. Grant Jr., *Black Men, Intergenerational Colonialism, and Behavioral Health*, https://doi.org/10.1007/978-3-030-21114-1_4

are influenced by social institutions, and their current behavior is constrained and incentivized by existing institutions" (Little, 2012, p. 4). This creates a fluid connectivity to anthropology that literally translates from Latin origins to mean the study of mankind, a discipline that works to explore the intersections of time, culture and geography across the globe.

According to Kurt Lewin, one of Social Psychology's founding fathers, the discipline is "a scientific means of fostering democratic, egalitarian norms and preventing tyranny and oppression from gaining the upper hand in society" (Jost & Kay, 2010, p. 1123). This description evidences the value of exploring the theoretical paradigms that afford academics and practitioners with the ability to address systemic risk factors and positively affect outcomes for people. Exploring the systems identified in the bio-ecological model of human development through the lens of historical trauma and contemporary oppression works to effectively disaggregate the often overwhelming context in which Black men have existed across generations in many Euronormative nations, particularly those identified in this study.

The value of theoretical exploration is limited absent an actionable framework that produces sustainable solution-driven paradigms, practices and policies. One of the most effective ways to reach this goal is the application of a public health lens to information gleaned through the analysis of data from tested theories and hypotheses. Public health is a scientific discipline that focuses on preventing deleterious conditions and outcomes by analyzing data from comprehensive sets of risk and protective factors influencing a group of people. The focus might be a small geographically proximate population of the public or a larger group spread across a wide swath of the globe who share a common ethnic heritage. The beauty of the public health model is that imbedded in its theoretical framework is a call to action that requires practitioners to act. Once the contributing factors are assessed, specific solution-based efforts are developed and implemented to positively impact community wellness, early intervention, equitable access and/or inclusive legislation.

Urie Bronfenbrenner, a Russian-born, Harvard-educated psychologist, concluded that the development of all individuals is reliant upon and responsive to a set of systems in which they exist. Although the individual's ability to manipulate many of these systems is limited, the system's impact on the individual is consistently significant. By the late 1980s, Bronfenbrenner's work had been widely researched and replicated by other psychologists and researchers in, what was then, the burgeoning field of Ecological Psychology. He called his theory the Bio-Ecological Model of Human Development, and it has been used to guide policy, inform practice and was even influential in the development of the American Head-Start education model.

During the 1964 State of the Union address, American President Lyndon B. Johnson declared a "War on Poverty". The observations warranting this action were wide and broad but largely grounded in research that spoke to a municipal government's responsibility to compensate for inequities that saturate social, academic and economic conditions. One major inequity was related to the kindergarten preparedness of youth impacted by poverty compared to those who were not. The American Head Start program was designed to break poverty cycles by providing pre-school children from under-resourced communities and families with programs to meet a holistic set of emotional, nutritional, intellectual and psychological needs that addressed the varied ecologies in which they existed.

Ecological Psychology explains how the five systems of the Bio-Ecological Model of Human Development interact in a bi-directional fashion to inform the development of the whole person across their lifespan. This discipline further identifies a set of environmental risk and protective categories that consistently and reliably support outcomes for most all people. The Bio-Ecological Model of Human Development associates five different systems in the outcomes of growth and development for all people. The most proximate system described in this theoretical model is the microsystem. The workplaces of adults, the classrooms of adolescents and the homes of infants all represent microsystems, systems in which individuals are directly immersed. Individuals experience this environment directly and on a daily basis. People's attitudes and behaviors are influenced by the characteristics of their microsystems and those systems' interactions with their unique genotypes and phenotypes. In a parallel and bi-directional process, one's microsystems are influenced by the behaviors the individual exhibits, the activities in which they engage and the attitudes they endorse. While this is happening, their microsystems are also acting upon each of those behaviors, activities and attitudes (Bronfenbrenner, 1994).

The quality of the relationships that families have with their child's school or that a caregiver has with their local community park is mediated by the mesosystem which links one's varied microsystems. The exosystem describes spaces individuals don't usually have influence over as exemplified by a child's inability to make decisions on the time their parents are allowed to leave their workplace. Workplaces that require long hours or consistently cut shifts without notice present serious risk factors to the child's microsystem in the same way that a well-paying job with paid sick leave introduces protections to their microsystem (Bronfenbrenner, 1994).

Each of the aforementioned systems is highly impacted by and impactful to the final two systems: the macrosystem and the chronosystem. The outer most layer of the concentric circles often used to represent the bio-ecological model of human development is the macrosystem. Laws, cultural norms and customs are macrosystemic components that all influence how each of the other systems works, both inter- and intrasystemically (Bronfenbrenner, 1994). If a municipality's macrosystem demonstrates a particular cultural affinity for older adults, its neighborhoods would house relevant community-based resources, its government would provide affordable housing in convenient locations and local resources would be allocated to the creation of programs that mitigate gaps due to decades of exponential technological advances. Similar resources would be dedicated to the eradication of risk factors that rendered the children of families in poverty less able to thrive across several domains if the ecological systems were reflective of their collective impact.

President Johnson was once a school teacher in a one-room school house in Texas and held a strong belief in the role that a successful education played in the dismantling of cycles and systems that maintained poverty. The experts who assembled to address his war on poverty came to some conclusions, and the Cooke Report was one of them. The Cooke Report of 1965 developed recommendations detailing how comprehensive education, health nutrition, social services and parent involvement plans could provide children experiencing disadvantage with a "head start". This "head start", informed by child development research, would address the inequities of poverty and the effects of food uncertainty and housing insecurity. In 1965, President Johnson announced the launch of Project Head Start, an eight-week summer program to serve over a half-million children and their families across the country. As a result of the summer programs' successes, Congress authorized the program to be expanded across a full nine-month period. Much of the research used to initiate the idea and create the Head Start program was from the Bio-Ecological Model of Human Development. The idea of the Head Start program met with success during a time when rectifying inequity and injustice were forefront. Each of these factors benefitted from a time system that afforded the freedom of thought and cognitive top-of-mindedness that resulted in deliberate and measurable efforts aimed at decreasing achievement gaps across several ecological domains (Udo-Akang, 2012; Vinovskis, 2005).

The final system that Bronfenbrenner described was the chronosystem. As its prefix indicates, the chronosystem is one shaped by the nuances of the specific time in which the identified development occurs (Bronfenbrenner, 1994). Chronosystem is often best explained through comparison across a specific construct. Bullying has been a part of the lives of school aged children for centuries. The nature, intensity and mechanisms of bullying, however, have devolved over time. The gravity of its consequences have also strengthened, but why and how? In the 1960s, many would agree that bullying ended at school dismissal. If caregivers never allowed a bully to enter the home, threats and violence wouldn't commence again until the next morning, providing survivors of bullying with a daily 15–16-hour respite from the perpetrators' malevolent provocations. Due to the contemporary chronosystemic features of relatively affordable cellular phone networks, moderately wide reaching internet access and egocentric social media platforms, bullying can technically impact an individual's complete set of microsystem engagements for 24 hours uninterrupted. It wouldn't be unusual to potentiate that increases in segments of youth suicides are due to chronosystemic factors that exponentially increase youth exposure to various traumas related to bullying in their microsystems. The situation is only worsened by the steady endorsement of these platforms across macrosystemic models that consistently violate civility.

Each of these systems looks different for different people. Even when the physical container and geographic space of the systems are identical (i.e. Children who grow up in the same home, adults who work for the same company or older adults who live in the same city), the permutations of outcomes are limitless. This is due to several factors, most notably the unique biology of each individual and the varied combinations of intersectionality in their bio-sociocultural identities. Current chronosystemic factors like contemporary oppression and discursive injury supplant themselves on multi-systemic components of historical trauma and Eurocentrism for Black men and boys across two continents. The remainder of this chapter explores the synergy created by these systemic engagements to detail the uniqueness held within the collective experiences and associated outcomes for Black men.

In 1965, Daniel Patrick Moynihan, a sociologist serving as Assistant Secretary of Labor for President Johnson, published a report entitled *The Negro Family: The Case for National Action*. Known more commonly as the Moynihan Report, it too was created as a part of Johnson's War on

Poverty. The report's aim was to address the multi-systemic conditions that impact Black people, specifically those at the intersection of race oppression and socio-economic depression. In the report, Moynihan details the key factors believed to impact the conditions experienced by Black Americans during the 1960s. Moynihan highlighted the importance of Black men gaining equitable access to jobs that create the opportunity to make meaningful contributions toward the support of their families. If this did not happen, he predicted the systematic alienation from their roles as fathers and husbands increasing the numbers of children developing without a biological father in spite of the parent's relationship status. This report is another example of the influences of environmental psychology research on policy and practice. Moynihan believed that jobs, vocational training and educational programs in the Black community would work to mediate the multi-systemic intergenerational factors responsible for the data he mined (Moynihan, 1965).

One of the most intriguing components of the bio-ecological model of human development is the bi-directional nature of influence that each system has over the other. The Moynihan Report was highly criticized for what some characterized as underlying messages that vilified Blackness. It was stated that this vilification occurred through an emphasis on the need for assimilation and integration as mechanisms to render one distant from their cultural traditions in exchange for the adoption of Euronormative value systems, value systems purported to result in wellness and positive outcomes. In his report, Moynihan describes the pervasiveness of racism in America was like a virus in a blood stream. He added, optimistically, that Black Americans would continue to encounter serious personal prejudice and racism for a minimum of one more generation. He stressed what he described as a national goal aimed at: the establishment of a stable "Negro family structure" by addressing how enslavement, Reconstruction, urbanization, unemployment and poverty serve as key underlying factors to the microsystemic concerns he described (Moynihan, 1965).

Both the Head Start Program and Moynihan's *The Negro Family: The Case for National Action* were born into the same exosystem promoted by a common macrosystem. They both took into account the manner in which intergenerational disadvantage contributed to the repetitious nature of these cyclic conditions. Although they were to be operationalized in mostly overlapping microsystems within the same chronosystem, Moynihan's report would not gain the support granted the Head Start program. There is no question that the lens through which his report was written left out those culturally empathic strength-based paradigms common in contemporary reports, but this example is a reflection of characteristics present in many Black microsystems of the time (Moynihan, 1965; Udo-Akang, 2012).

Black microsystems across the diaspora grew a connectedness surrounding half a decade of significant chronosystemic events. The experiences within these microsystems resulted in a force that predictably influenced the reception of Moynihan's report by the Black community. By 1966, the Emancipation Proclamation and the Thirteenth Amendment to the Constitution were just a century old. In 1960, the North Carolina A&T Four had staged their sit-in at the segregated Woolworths counter in Greensboro, and John F. Kennedy had been elected US President. Dr. Martin Luther King Jr. delivered his *I Have a Dream* speech in 1963 just before the passing of the Civil Rights Act of 1964 and the Voting Rights Act of 1965, each major reference points in the Civil Rights Movement. Pan Africanism began to grow as Algeria gained independence from France in 1962 and the Organization of African Unity—currently the African Union—was formed in 1963. Both Malcolm X and John F. Kennedy were assassinated in 1965 just before Kwanzaa held its first celebration and the Black Power Movement was organized in 1966.

The condition created at the intersection of the 1960's American chronosystem and Black microsystems rendered interpretations of the Moynihan Report's intentions antithetical to how Black men and women were experiencing themselves. In 1961, Dr. Martin Luther King Jr., in reference to the existential space of Black people in this new chronosystem, stated: "The new militancy grew out of the Negro's growing sense of dignity and destiny. Whenever people get a new sense of dignity they become more determined to do away with the barriers to freedom" (Levingston, 2017, p. 42). The events in the 1960s coalesced into a space where Black consciousness had evolved from seeking liberty to demanding equity. These microsystemic experiences generated responses aimed at the exosystem's efforts to inflict what seemed like very familiar traumatic injury, one born from a history of paternalistic domination and efforts of forced assimilation.

Trauma

The Diagnostic and Statistical Manual of Mental Disorders 5th ed. (DSM-V) describes trauma as exposure to actual or threatened death, serious injury, or sexual violence ... (by) directly experiencing the traumatic event(s); witnessing, in person, the traumatic event(s) as it occurred to others, learning that the traumatic event(s) occurred to a close family member or close friend ... or experiencing repeated or extreme exposure to aversive details of the traumatic event(s). (American Psychiatric Association, 2013)

Within each chronosystem of development from the commencement of early European colonialism and imperialism, Black men and boys as a group, when compared to other men and boys, have disproportionately been exposed to both subjective and objective race-based traumatic stimuli. Discussing these experiences in isolation fails to adequately honor the totality or gravity of the ecosystemic settings that disproportionately distributes the benefits and burdens of the societies in which they develop. These experiences are not sufficiently explored absent the content experienced by the prior generations and contexts into which the generations to follow were born.

Historical, transgenerational, intergenerational and collective trauma have all been used interchangeably alongside post-colonial distress throughout research. Although they are not all synonymous, they share an important underlying spirit that illustrates how the experiences of one's ancestors influence current systems and the individuals in them in a very real way. The concept of historical trauma as it relates to the post-colonial experiences of Indigenous people in North America first appeared in behavioral health literature in the mid-1990s. Research from the existing frameworks of historical oppression and psychological trauma were framed together to contextualize "Indigenous health problems as forms of post-colonial suffering, to de-stigmatize Indigenous individuals whose recovery was thwarted by paralyzing self-blame, and to legitimate Indigenous cultural practices as therapeutic interventions in their own right" (Kirmayer, Gone, & Moses, 2014, p. 300). Historical trauma differs from other types of trauma due to these intergenerational qualities. It has been used to explain many of the behavioral health disparities among Indigenous populations and First Nations People across the world, from Australia to the USA and Canada. This wide body of research regarding American Indian, First Nations and Aboriginal populations states that:

the trauma of the loss of land, culture, and people has never been resolved, but has been anesthetized by alcohol and other drugs. Native American people suffer from post-traumatic stress disorder as a consequence of the devastating effects of genocide perpetrated by the US government. (Gone, 2014, pp. 388–389)

All men of African descent have at least one common historical thread that binds them, that of enslavement and European colonialism. Even if one's biological ancestors had never been enslaved, this experience is a collective one impacting a peoplehood due to its scope and magnitude. This occurs in the same way that the entire diaspora of Jewish people experience ramifications of the Holocaust, even if their families escaped persecution or were never knowledgeably in harm's way. Kirmayer et al. (2014) define historical trauma using what they refer to as the "The Four C's": *Colonial Injury* by European settlers who perpetuate conquest and subjugation, a *collective experience* of these injuries by groups whose identities and relationships were fractured as a consequence, the *cumulative effects* from the injuries facilitated and catalyzed by "sequences of adverse policies and practices" and the *cross generational* impacts of these injuries as "legacies of risk and vulnerability were passed from ancestors to descendants". Disenfranchised grief, internalized oppression and historical unresolved grief are additional factors that researchers have included in the cadre of psycho-sociocultural factors associated with historical trauma (Brave-Heart, 2014). These factors create a clear and concise heptagonal container in which historical trauma manifests itself.

Evidence from the mitochondrial DNA (mtDNA) genome shows that many Black men across the globe share a common genetic, geographic and contextual ancestry, creating a geno-historically linked group (Salas, Carrecedo, Richard, & Macaulay, 2005; Schroeder et al., 2015). Mitochondrial DNA is used as a tool for research across disciplines from anthropology and phylogenetics to biogeography and forensic sciences. It is also often used to trace genetic lineage as it exists through maternal ancestry. While the vast majority of our genetic code is found inside cell nuclei where our nuclear DNA (nDNA) lives, mtDNA is found in energy-producing cell organelles known as mitochondria. In addition to location and number of molecules in a given cell, mtDNA and nDNA differ in several other ways. Mitochondrial DNA is circular in form, is unable to independently produce the full catalog of life-sustaining proteins, hosts fewer DNA base pairs, is not easily subject to recombination and is highly preserved over time (Chial & Craig, 2008; Salas et al., 2005).

"The Atlantic slave trade promoted by West European empires (fifteenth–nineteenth centuries) forcibly moved at least 11 million people from Africa, including one-third from west-central Africa to European and American destinations" (Salas et al., 2005, p. 676). Studies using mtDNA to trace lineage appears to identify West Africa, south western Africa and west-central Africa as the geographic origins of men and women of African descent across the Americas and Caribbean. East and Southeast Africa are poorly represented in the mtDNA occurrences in North American populations of people of African descent (Salas et al., 2005; Schroeder et al., 2015). Slavery took the indigenous African and displaced him and his family based on constructs of European superiority. The events that resulted in the collective extraction and enslavement of generations of Africans created a colonial injury that persisted for 400 years.

The institution of slavery was based upon the thought that indigenous people of color throughout the world were in need of civilizing. Although this value system was grounded in a common long-held belief in a biological predisposition that made these groups sub-human, it would take centuries for it to be published as academic research. In the late 1700s, Johann Blumenbach, a German anthropologist, developed the hierarchy of difference, a system of classifying people predicated upon socially constructed ideas of superior and inferior races. In this hierarchy, people of European descent were at the top while people of African descent were on the bottom. European scholars, anthropologist and colonialists studied, labeled and categorized non-Whites and created literature attesting to their inferiority while implicitly and explicitly inscribing their own White European superiority (Sorrells, 2016). The art, literature, research and assessment tools throughout history were informed and influenced by this theory to create an ecology shared by every Black man without reference to the specific geographical space he inhabits or the enslavement status of his ancestors.

Blumenbach's theory resulted in several other bodies of research that catalyzed ideologies relegating Blacks to the lowest station across several domains. The hereditarian position states that genetics and heritability play significant roles in behavioral traits such as personality, criminality and intelligence and is responsible for both the contexts and constructs in which contemporary Black men exist. In the 1800s, theories on race-based intelligence and criminality dominated the English Victorian literature and pseudo-science. Aristotle, Voltaire, Rousseau, David Hume and many others published works that discussed the genetic inferiority of the "Negro"

(Robinson, 2000; Rushton, 1997). In the 1840s, a Spanish doctor, named in the literature only by Soler, made one of the first references to the born criminal (Gabbidon & Taylor, 2012). European explorers even wrote upon contact that "Africans have a very low intelligence and few words to express complex thoughts" (Rushton, 1997). In 1849, Italian Army Doctor Cesare Lombrosso published *The Criminal Man* which suggested a causal link between race and crime (Gabbidon & Taylor, 2012). It wasn't unusual for people to purport the heritability of socially harmful traits like pauperism, criminality and mental illness, particularly as it related to Black people. In 1883, scientist Francis Galton coined the term Eugenics to highlight the value in providing the "more suitable" races with opportunities for success compared to those deemed less suitable for success (Sussman, 2014). This theoretical foundation was being spread and crystallized in the same chronosystem where intelligence tests were being developed in Europe and exported to America.

The first Intelligence tests were developed by French psychologist Alfred Binet and subsequently brought to America in 1880 by American psychologist, Henry Goddard. A prominent hereditarian and US psychologist, Lewis Ternman introduced the term Intelligence Quotient (IQ) to the US lexicon based on the 1912 research of German psychologist Lewis Stern. By the 1920s, Eugenics "commanded the support of most Euro-American intellectuals" (Sussman, 2014). The American Eugenics Society even praised Hitler in 1933 for his sterilization laws. Contemporary oppression is built upon a strong foundation of historically traumatic events impacting generations of citizens globally victimized by the pseudo-science of racial inferiority. This collection of thought and theory culminates in a cacophony of justifications to further oppress Black people, justifications including but not limited to psychological, academic, behavioral and criminogenic factors. The collective attributional errors, stereotypes, oppressive laws, acts of psychological terrorism, events of political violence and physical abuses create a synergistic effect that results in outcomes much larger than would exist if each of these risk factors were independently present (Sussman, 2014).

Trauma Transmission

For many, what is most challenging to understand is not the actual components that make up historical trauma, but the apparatus responsible for cross generational impact ensuring that each age band of a particular group inherits the injury and its associated symptoms. Coyle (2014) indicated that untreated trauma in a parent might be transmitted to the child through the level of security associated with the attachment bond and/or the messages sent about the child's self-identity and safety or danger inherent in the environments where they live. Collective injuries that occur over time to people who share a specific affiliation like ethnicity, affectional orientation or religion have the capacity to impact generations of that group who never experienced the injurious events. The political violence experienced by Black people is remembered and recounted regularly to other Blacks who are currently experiencing the events that will be the content of their future narratives of unresolved political violence. Such experiences and memories in totality play a significant role on the ways in which one experiences helplessness, optimism, grief or success. They are all influenced by that individual's perception of the world reflected through ones sense of self. Kellerman (2008) demonstrates how four cross-disciplinary theoretical orientations explain the transmission of trauma across generations.

Table 4.1, adapted from Kellerman's work, summarizes the transmission factors discussed.

Psychodynamic theory describes trauma transmission through how children take on the repressed emotional experiences their parents were unable to manage or even consciously experience at all. Projective identification is a psychoanalytic mechanism of trauma transmission hypothesized as a means of coping with the lasting effects of political violence. "Parents who have suffered from political violence may use projective identification for the purposes of self-healing, unconsciously using their children as a means to psychic recovery" (Weingarten, 2004, p. 14). Black parents of Black adolescent males, most of whom have either experienced political violence or been impacted by historical trauma, are subject to project intolerable beliefs and ideas about themselves onto their children.

Table 4.1 Transmission model of historical trauma (Kellerman, 2008)

Theory	Transmission apparatus	Main factors transmitted
Psychodynamic	Interpersonal relationships	Unconscious displaced emotion
Socio-cultural	Socialization	Parenting and role models
Family systems	Communication	Enmeshment
Biological	Genetic	Hereditary vulnerability to PTSD

A Black father who grew up in the 1960s might suffer significant psychic damage due to experiences with extreme racism, institutional disenfranchisement and legalized discrimination. This father is likely to pass an array of his unendurable fears about himself and his perceptions of agency on to his son. Early on, the son, without awareness, takes on these fears. Projective identification can be enacted by family members rapidly, can occur outside of conscious awareness and can inspire children to tap into a variety of pro- and anti-social relational work to repair experiences suffered by their parents. "When the parents use of projective identification is excessive, it has severe implications for the whole of the child's psychic development" (Silverman & Lieberman, 1999, p. 1). Socio-cultural theory provides a context where traumas are transmitted through social norms, beliefs, taboos and fears. This theory's transmission method illustrates an unconscious yet direct effect of parents' behaviors on their children.

Familial mechanisms focus on family life which provides an infinite number of permutations for the transmission of intergenerational trauma. Family Systems theory determines that both verbal and non-verbal parental communication patterns encourage enmeshment by unintentionally or intentionally discouraging individuation. This communication pattern may be attributed to and informed by the parent/caregiver's challenges related to the historical traumas that they have experienced, knowingly or not. There are severe challenges to modeling empowered communication when the models themselves have been strategically disempowered over time. A major goal of parents, in relation to their children, is protection. The provision of warnings for dangers that lie in wait for Black boys that look different from any of their counterparts. In recent years, Black families have openly discussed what has been referred to as "The Talk". The Talk is a non-discrete dissemination of information and tools to Black boys over time to arm them as their innocence is systematically broken across the duration of their lifespan through late adolescence. As parents approach these discussions, it is triggering for them as the information being shared to secure safety is a part of the narrative that awakens past traumatic experiences of their own, their parents and their parent's parents.

Caregivers often employ a less clear form of communication concerning the cultural trauma or political violence they experience(d). "They may not literally tell an anecdote, but symbolically communicate the message in other ways. Or the parent may have decided not to speak about experiences but rather responses to stimuli that remind him or her of the experience may provide a 'map' to what he or she has suffered"

(Weingarten, 2004, p. 17). In these instances, meanings about trauma are miscommunicated and children are left to their own interpretation. Children are known to be astute observers. If they witness, learn of or feel that parents or grandparents have been humiliated, they become vulnerable to the development of "retaliatory fantasies". They watch the ways adults react and use emotions during these varied situations and create their own emotional responsivity to the situation while noting the continuum of behaviors that accompany those responses. Young adults might adapt their behavior according to these cues as they move across their stages of development. "The transgenerational transmission of such a shared traumatic event is linked to the past generation's inability to mourn losses of people, land or prestige, and indicated the large group's failure to reverse … humiliation inflicted by another large group" (Volcan, 2001, p. 87). Black youth of each generation bear the burden of redemption for the history of violence and brutality that impacted each generation of their forefathers since the commencement of African enslavement.

Other models describing the transgenerational transmission of historical trauma employ a wider web of cooperation, integration and bi-directional interaction between the activities and events at the national, community, family and individual levels. The following assertions are applied to each nation in this study. Data demonstrates that Black men across every post-enslavement generation throughout Canada, the USA, the UK and France have been—and continue to be—exposed to several transgenerational transmission factors at each level. Each nation compels—through extreme power—the forced assimilation of Black men in an aim to eliminate a sense of collective identification. The eradication of collective identity for Black men is rarely researched across international borders. Even more neglected are the intra-nationally sanctioned and facilitated divisions that create tension and strife between Black men who share post-colonial national identities. The loss of collective identity attaches itself to an environment where eugenic and genocidal patterns of behavior and legislation continue to thrive under these nation's agendas.

Finally, a highly maintained system of national exclusion has created a gaping hole of voicelessness for Black people in these nations. The consistent and overwhelmingly vast political leadership of White men across the globe remains striking. The European Union (EU) was created after World War II to foster a sense of economic cooperation and trade among the countries. It began in the 1950s as the European Economic Community (EEC) with six countries and has grown to now represent 28. The EU is governed by the European Commission—officially known as the College—on which each member country has a representative whose aim is enhancement of the EU as a whole and not their individual national interests. This group, led by its president and five vice presidents, makes decisions, proposes laws, funds programs and determines budgets. The College has a huge degree of influence over the direction of the EU, and as of 2018, each of its commissioners was White (Rankin, 2018).

The EU as a body addresses and determines a wide range of guidelines and procedures including but not limited to research and training, agriculture, the environment and transportation. The EU is divided into four separate institutions: The European Commission, the European Parliament, the Council of the European Union and the Court of Justice. Equitable representation of Blacks as Members of European Parliament (MEP's) would be 22, around 3%. The European Parliament is comprised of 751 members, and only 3 are Black, which is less than a half of a percent (Rankin, 2018). At their founding in 1992, the EU would also define the factors rendering one a European Citizen. This citizenship provided details for individuals who were already citizens of the Member States—by naturalization or birthright—on rules related to movement between countries, consular protection when abroad and participation in the European Parliament. The spirit of the European citizenship paradigm was to complement national citizenship and not replace it.

Researchers and observers have been consistently reflective on the challenges with the EU's attention to race and diversity. It is widely known that EU institutions collect data on an array of staff demographics, including nationality, age and gender … but not on race or ethnicity. Although this is not uncommon in European countries—in France, it remains illegal to collect race data on citizens—it serves as a true barrier to definitively understand and document whether progress toward racial equity is or isn't occurring across Member States. The European Network Against Racism (ENAR), established by grassroots activists in 1998, is a Pan-European anti-racism network created to generate continental legal changes regarding racism and make decisive progress toward racial equality. The lens through which ENAR achieves this is through addressing and ending structural racism and discrimination across Europe and effect real change in the lives of ethnic and religious minorities. ENAR representatives have been outspoken about the EU's seemingly consistent policy of ignoring and even burying issues of race as a strategy to passively address the growing concerns (European Network Against Racism (ENAR)).

The EU's 2017 Diversity and Inclusion Charter (European Commission, 2017) originally came under fire due to its notable silence on issues of discrimination related to racial minorities. The EU's diversity charter represents a commitment of the European Commission's efforts toward equal treatment and opportunities for all. It is dedicated to the inclusion of all European citizens "irrespective of … sex, race, colour, ethic or social origin, genetic features, language, religion or belief, political or any other opinion, the membership of a national minority, property, birth, disability, age or sexual orientation" (European Commission, 2017, p. 1).

As a result of policies supporting forced assimilation, generations of youth are left without a fluid model or mechanism through which positive ethnic identity development might occur. This is due in part to the deficits-based paradigms that perpetuate stereotyping and negative imagery of Black communities and those it is comprised of. Within these communities, the external promotion of disorganization, conflict and social problems support a self-fulfilling prophecy where identity is patterned after paternalistic archetypes born of and buttressed by systems of structural oppression.

Communities are composed of families and individuals who often reflect the conditions of their varied microsystems. These reflections—for some—show a beautiful set of outcomes that echo environments supportive of optimal functioning at both the familial and individual levels. For others, these reflections result in reverberations of grief, learned helplessness, abuse and dysfunction, oftentimes independent of socio-economic status. As families approach the crossroads to or to not reconcile these experiences, they model—to youth and one another—one of the many severe microsystemic consequences of oppression. This is in addition to supremacy's propensity to thrive across the lifespan and travel across generations. At the individual level, these experiences and conditions are known to facilitate environments that trigger symptoms of mental health ailments, challenges in nuclear family dyads, low self-esteem and impaired identity development. In a very obvious way, these individual factors work bi-directionally to exacerbate family dysfunction and community disorganization. The aim is to ensure that ancestral wounds remain unhealed as they are germane to the maintenance of contemporary systems of oppression.

In 1935, the Belgian colonial government introduced group classification ID cards to Rwandan communities. The colonial power took control of the country and its neighbor Burundi during World War I in the mid-1920s. Prior to Belgium's policy on direct colonial rule, the countries were—as a result of the Berlin Conference—under the auspices of Germany whose comparative laissez faire approach ruled through the existing Rwandan monarchy. The ID card labeled each individual, most of whom were native Rwandan, as Tutsi, Hutu, Twa or Naturalized. The Belgian colonial forces ruled in a fashion that deepened the divide between the Hutu and Tutsi, further disenfranchising the Hutu. This pattern was continued from the eighteenth-century Tutsi domination and nineteenth-century land expansion. The Hutu were the country's population majority but were experiencing severe disenfranchisement. Although contemporary archaeology and paleoanthropology link the Hutu and Tutsi to the original Bantu Expansion, both the Germans and the Belgians believed the Hutu were an inferior group deserving of suppression from the Tutsi who they believed had fewer indigenous African features when compared to the Hutu. Many Europeans believed that the Tutsi were descendants of the Hamites who were thought to represent an African-European admixture. The criteria for initial Belgian classification defined Tutsi as anyone who either had more than ten cows or favored phenotypic characteristics like a longer nose or neck (Dallaire, 2015; Mamdani, 2002).

After World War II, the Hutu Social Movement was formed to fight for equality and against oppression. European sentiment had also begun to shift resulting in many Belgians in support of equity for the Hutu people. The Hutu, who had been marginalized and disenfranchised through a system exploited by colonial rule, were now empowered. After decades of support from the Belgian military to suppress the Hutus, the Belgian government would now support a Hutu leader after the Tutsi government was overthrown and thousands of Tutsi Rwandans were forced to neighboring lands. In 1990, those Tutsi refugees would return home under the Rwandan Patriotic Front to challenge the Hutu government. This would result in the Rwandan Civil War which began in 1990. The war would end with Rwanda being forced to navigate a system of Hutu–Tutsi shared governance after decades of colonial reliance on a system that deepened divisions and crystallized hatred. In 1994, Hutu President Juvénal Habyarimana's plane was shot down killing all passengers on board. The civil war had ended less than a year before, and the country found itself again immersed in violent warfare (Dallaire, 2015; Mamdani, 2002).

With the aim of cleansing the country of political opposition and avoiding a future of potential subjugation, the Hutu launched a genocidal attack on the Tutsi population of Rwanda. Hutu civilians were armed with machetes and other weapons and compelled to kill their neighbors, rape their wives and steal their land. It is estimated that 800,000 people died in this genocide which accounted for the obliteration of 70% of the Tutsi population. In less than a three-month period, hundreds of thousands were murdered in hand-to-hand community-based combat, mostly with machetes and short range firearms. Reports of subsequent race-based genocidal events continued throughout the late 1990s in the forms of Tutsi bus passengers being murdered at a road block outside the capitol, 39 Rwandan's being burned alive on a bus in Rubavu or 6 children murdered at the Nyange Secondary school (Dallaire, 2015; Mamdani, 2002).

In 1996, Athanase Hagengimana, a native Rwandan psychiatrist and researcher, conducted a door-to-door interview survey of families in communities in and surrounding the Rwandan capital of Kigali. Using the Kinyarwanda translation of the Harvard Trauma Questionnaire and Standardized Psychiatric Interview, the former medical school vice dean found that slightly over 50% of the 157 respondents met DSM-IV criteria for a diagnosable psychiatric disorder. The genocide left hundreds of thousands dead, and one of the only published research studies of the time demonstrated that half of the remaining population was impacted by a diagnosable psychiatric condition that included acute grief reaction, depression and PTSD. Such a high prevalence of a diagnosable disorder is considered a public health epidemic warranting intervention and evidence-informed insight as to what that means for the future of individual communities and the country at large (Hagengimana, Hinton, Bird, Pollack, & Pitman, 2003).

Epigenetic research has demonstrated that the glucocorticoid receptor exon 1F promoter can be modulated by stressors from the environment and might impact one's vulnerability and resilience to psychiatric disorders. In 2012, researchers in the Democratic Republic of the Congo found that maternal stress was correlated with both low birth weight and increased methylation of the glucocorticoid receptor gene in 25 mother-newborn dyads (Youssef, Lockwood, Su, Hao, & Rutten, 2018). Researchers who authored a study published in a 2014 issue of the *World Journal of Biological Psychiatry* sought to discover the impact of the Tutsi genocide on children of women who were pregnant in Rwanda during the genocide. The study entitled, "The Tutsi genocide and transgenerational transmission of maternal stress: epigenetics and biology of the HPA axis" (Peroud et al., 2014), assessed the DNA of 50 Rwandan women and their children. Twenty-five of the women were widows who were pregnant in Rwanda during the genocide, while the remaining (the control group), also of Rwandan origin and pregnant during the genocide, lived outside of Rwanda during their pregnancies. The mothers and children exposed to the genocide not only exhibited higher rates of PTSD and depression and lower cortisol levels (associated with PTSD) when compared to the control group, they also showed higher methylation levels at exon 1F promoter suggesting that trauma-induced methylation changes in humans can be passed from parent to biological offspring. Although the discussion of mechanisms responsible for the transmission of trauma across generations heretofore has focused on psychological and socio-cultural factors, this research supports the existence of bio-genetic factors that serve as transmission mechanisms working in concert with the others (Peroud et al., 2014). Most all human behaviors and experiences are guided and informed by factors generated from activities occurring in genes. How these genes engage with and respond to their internal environment (initiation of protein production, transcription, apoptosis, etc.) and how they are or are not modified due to stimuli from the external environment (methylation, chromatid remodeling, etc.) tell the story of each individual's life course.

Epigenetics is defined as the development of established changes in DNA expression not attributable to mutations or sequence alterations. It is a demonstration of how environmental, chemical and physical dynamics affect, transform and pass down a genotype's set of phenotypic expressions. Epigenetic factors operationalize themselves through the upregulation or downregulation of the gene as a result of external stimuli like nutritious vitamins, psychological anxiety, stress and environmental pollutants. Epigenetic modulations like psychological state, financial status, disease exposure, substance abuse, diet and quality of social interactions all impact how our genes work (Peroud et al., 2014).

Methylation, the second most frequently occurring chemical reaction in the human body, is largely responsible for determining if and when genes are regulated up or down. The process itself uses methyl groups also known as hydrocarbons to support a population's ability to respond to environmental and ecological changes. Methylation is required to change a variety of enzymes into forms the body is able to use. As the large hydrocarbons attach to the promoter genes, they block transcription factors from being able to copy the gene with the fidelity known to optimize outcomes of gene expression. What's copied is a compromised nuclear characteristic that represses or silences a gene that is now rendered heritable as newly reproduced cells within the organism itself or in the organism's progeny, including humans and other vertebrate mammals. Choline, folic acid and vitamin B12 are all methyl group nutrients that produce positive health outcomes during pre-natal care, child development and aging across the lifespan. Methyl groups are attracted to areas of DNA to stop the presentation of the diseases that would be produced absent the blockage. When individuals have methylation deficiencies (either acquired or genetic), the likelihood of somatic and psychological dysfunctions like ADD, allergies, birth defects, schizophrenia, heart disease, infertility, hypertension, arthritis and cancer can increase (Babu & Banerjee, 2017; Beach et al., 2013; Hamza et al., 2017; Peroud et al., 2014; Youssef et al., 2018).

Histone modification is another mechanism by which epigenetics impact gene behavior without changing the actual DNA sequence. Histones are the proteins that make up the intracellular chromatin complexes used for the efficient packaging of DNA and RNA. When well organized and bundled, the infinitely long DNA and RNA sequence strands operate with a higher degree of efficiency. There are certain environmental conditions, like with methylation, that influence how proficient chromatin's molecular scaffolding is at supporting our nuclear material and optimizing its performance. The process of histone acetylation, for example, loosens the chromatin complex allowing increased access to nuclear material for replication and transcription, changes the interactions between histones in adjacent nucleosomes while doing the same to the relationship between regulatory proteins and histones. Other processes result in etherochromatin which increases the density of the complexes, compacting the nuclear material around the histones. This decreases accessibility and represses replication and transcription. Histone modification is also impacted by methylation as chromatin remodeling exposes nuclear segments that might have historically remained unexposed and vice versa (Babu & Banerjee, 2017; Beach et al., 2013; Hamza et al., 2017; Peroud et al., 2014; Youssef et al., 2018).

Like the 100 days of the Rwandan Genocide or the decade of the Jewish Holocaust, Black Americans experienced a discrete event marked by extraordinarily barbaric trauma. Unlike many other groups, Black men and women continued to experience a consistently evolving assault against their personhood, making it such that each generation continues to be granted experiences with their own personalized acute traumatic event. These generational events (enslavement, buck breaking, peonage, convict leasing, prison industrial complex) have the ability to impact the functioning of DNA sequences that have already been impacted generation over generation with pre-existing traumatic methylation and remodeled chromatin structures. Recent research speaks to the capacity for the injuries of racism and discrimination that may not rise to traumatic levels to cause epigenetic changes. People who did experience racial discrimination were found to have more methylation on the genes affecting schizophrenia, bipolar disorder and asthma than those whose lived experience did not include discrimination (Babu & Banerjee, 2017; Beach et al., 2013; Hamza et al., 2017; Peroud et al., 2014; Youssef et al., 2018).

Although research has found statistically significant correlations between human epigenetic changes associated with war trauma, genocide, intimate partner violence and child maltreatment, there remains a great deal of unrevealed knowledge in the field. The future of epigenetic research includes longitudinal studies, comparisons of developmental stages where traumatic experiences occur and attention to differences attributable to the source tissue from which the DNA is extracted. Many of the studies hold a range of acknowledged limitations that are likely to be explored well throughout the coming decades alongside those ecological risk factors that create new compounding injuries through tools of contemporary oppressive forces.

Contemporary Oppression

Canada saw its first ever racial discrimination trial in 1955 in the small Ontario community of Dresden, ironically the home of Josiah Henson, the man from whom Harriet Beecher Stowe's main character, Uncle Tom, was created. At the time, the population of Dresden was just over 2000 residents and 12% Afro-Canadian. Children attended the same schools and rode the same buses, yet there were establishments that continued to deny service to Black Canadians. Hugh Burnett, a local resident, lobbied against these practices but was consistently denied. The Canadian climate at best minimized the extent of racial animus and at worst denied any existence of racial discrimination. Even in 1954, after Canada passed the Fair Accommodation Practices Act making discrimination based on race, nationality or place of origin illegal, business owners in Dresden continued to refuse service to Black residents.

Oppression is the undue use of authority and/or power in a burdensome, cruel or unjust manner and typically manifests itself across both institutional and social domains. The Latin origin comes from the word "opprimere" meaning "to press down". Institutional oppression occurs when formal or covert restrictions from a powerful entity (i.e. municipal government, school system, judicial structure, military, etc.) are placed upon a group so that they may be abused and less able to compete with other social groups (Babu & Banerjee, 2017). The oppressed group subsequently experiences devaluation and deprivation of privileges by the empowered group. Social Oppression describes a relationship in which the "dominant group benefits from the systematic abuse, exploitation and injustice directed toward the subordinate group" (Javaid & Choi, 2017). The synergy between institutionally and socially oppressive forces is far greater than the sum of their individual components as illustrated in Dresden and across the American South with government's refusal to hold individual proprietors accountable to the new civil rights laws of the land outlawing race-based discrimination.

Contemporary oppression might be operationalized in municipal laws, disparate application of rules, social norms, dominant cultural practices or media exploitation, each of which has disenfranchised men of African descent across the globe across each generation. Each of these factors contributes significantly to dangerous outcomes in Black communities across the globe that directly impact Black men and boys and the families in which they exist. These factors create, catalyze or exacerbate inexcusable inequities in academia, employment, housing, medical care and poverty (Kirmayer et al., 2014).

Contemporary oppression was isolated as a variable because historically oppressive factors forced upon men of African descent are well articulated within the framework and throughout the literature of Historic Trauma. Each historical trauma has clear etiological connections to oppression and the existence of unequal systems of injustice. Contemporary oppression references institutional practices and social mores that are a part of history's living memory measured according to current human lifespans. Contemporary history often refers to the history remembered by most people alive (Catterall, 1997). Events that have occurred since the middle of the nineteenth century are typically included in what might be defined as "contemporary" at the time of this publication.

Contemporary oppression rears its head in a variety of forms, some expected and others less so. In 2014, a pastry shop in Auxerre, France, was compelled to change the name of their "Bamboula" pastries after public outcry. In 2017, an ice cream maker in Nivelles, a French-speaking city in Belgium, also served a treat by the same name and as a result of social media self-advocacy, a disgusted patron forced the company to change the treat's name. Bamboula, a derogatory term whose etymology is of an African instrument, currently connotes an over-sexualized cannibalistic wild African man (Papirblat, 2017). In the 1980s, a different bakery in Belgium was forced by customers to rename the Bamboula cookies they were selling, yet the family-owned ice cream company and the Auxerre bakery seemed to have been unaware that their pastries might be insulting an entire group of citizens. In 2015, a court in the French Riviera ordered a French pastry shop to stop selling chocolate pastries reminiscent of colonial and slave trade images of the past. Even after being told by Black French citizens that the gingerbread pastries, covered in dark chocolate with extraordinarily exaggerated genitalia and minstrel show-style eyes and lips, were offensive, the baker, Tannick Tavolaro, continued to produce and display them (*The Local*, 2015).

The scope, frequency and impact of contemporary race oppression in Europe has been minimized throughout each chronosystem ever since a numerable population of non-immigrant Black European men have called France and Britain home. When race incidences are so often compared to American statistics, it tends to cloak the dangerous disproportionality and racially charged existence reported by Black people in these nations through their own narratives. By the end of the twentieth century, anti-discrimination bureaus in the Netherlands were registering an average of 3000 complaints per year. In its year of inception, the Commission Nationale Consultative des Droits de l'Homme, a French government hotline set up to assist survivors of discrimination, was overwhelmed with almost 14,000 calls in the first five months. That's over 93 calls per day, every day for five months to a system that had never before existed. During this same time, the British police reported over 47,000 "racial incidences", of which over 20,000 were crimes like assault, vandalism, harassment and wounding (Bleich, 2003).

Race policies are strategies and approaches aimed at mediating and managing the challenges of racism and relationships across cultural boundaries in diverse societies. Although Britain and France co-identify as models of political savviness and structural efficacy across the European Union, when it comes to race and ethnicity, their political paradigms couldn't be more different. France has adopted a nationwide color blind approach to governing and engaging its citizens while Britain uses data on race and ethnicity to make decisions and craft policies.

The French Constitution reads that "France shall be an indivisible, secular, democratic and social republic. It guarantees equality before the law for all citizens without distinction of origin, race or religion". In 2012, Socialist French presidential candidate François Hollande vowed to remove the word race from the constitution because from his point of view race doesn't exist and should thereby not be included in any official text (Diallo, 2018).

France has the largest population of Blacks in all of Europe but no ethnic statistics in the national census, although the law allows researchers and statisticians to collect such data as long as the subjects remain anonymous and the data is used for a study. After World War II, France, like many other nations, saw an immigration boom. People moving from North Africa, sub-Saharan Africa and South-East Asia to work in the economic boom of France settled, and had families, French families (Bleich, 2001). In 1972, France passed what has been referred to as their anti-racist laws and policies. These laws contain four major elements. It bans hate speech that provokes racial animus or violence, and it outlaws discrimination in employment or in the provision of goods and services. It allows the state to ban groups who promote racism, and it created a legal pathway for non-governmental anti-racist agencies to participate in court cases of racism as "civil parties" (Bleich, 2001). In 1978, the "Informatique et Libertés" was enacted which prohibited "except for exhaustively enumerated exceptions" the collection and recording of information that directly or indirectly identifies an individual's race, ethnicity or religion. Violation to this law is punishable by five years' imprisonment and a fine of €300,000 (Papirblat, 2017).

Conseil Representatif des Associations (CRAN) is a self-described anti-racist and anti-colonial group launched in 2005 to fight against the discrimination suffered by Black populations in France. Their foci address racism, social inequities and post-colonial injustices. Dr. Louis-George Tin, one of CRAN's founders, commissioned a private research study in 2008 to estimate the number of Blacks living in France. The study estimated that 1.8 million people in France were Black, representing an estimated 3% of the nation (Sorrells, 2016). The sample size, however, was so small (approximately 13,000 people) that it may not have been a good predictor of the actual Black population in the country. Other estimates place the Black French population at closer to 5%

with most being descendants from former French colonies across Africa and the Caribbean (Leduc & Frosch, 2013). The Paris-based National Consultative Commission on Human Rights (CNCDH) released a report that demonstrated a 23% increase in racist, anti-Semitic and anti-Muslim acts in 2012. Unfortunately, Frances' model of citizenship disenfranchises its Black citizens largely by allowing systems of structural inequality and their detrimental ramifications to grow unmeasured and untethered (Stille, 2014).

By 1966, the UK estimated that over 900,000 of their residents were "coloured". Less than 30 years later, 47% of the total ethnic minority population in the UK were native born citizens. During this same decade, the French census counted 700,000 immigrants of African and Asian descent but failed to count the country's citizens of color born in mainland France (Bleich, 2001). In 2016, the population of metropolitan France, not including its overseas territories, was 64.7 million people. Britain established the Commission for Racial Equality (CRE) which works on national campaigns against discrimination, produces annual reports on racism, provides financial support for organizations that fight racism and appraises organizations and industries that might be engaged in discriminatory business and hiring practices (Bleich, 2001).

Although both countries have outlawed many of the same racist crimes, Britain and France approach race adjudication differently as well. In France, punishments for racist crimes move through the criminal system, while in the UK they move through the civil system where the burden of proof is less of a risk factor to the delivery of justice. In 1991, it was reported that British civil courts saw over 1400 cases of employment discrimination where France's conviction of this same matter was only four (Bleich, 2001). According to policy research, France, in spite of its color blind approach, has adopted laws and practices that address racism and disparity through a geographic and socio-economic lens. The principal elements that ground France's national institutions include bans on hate speech, provocation of racial animus or violence, employment discrimination and groups supporting racism. In 1990, the Gayssot Law was passed. It expanded the 1972 anti-racists policies by adding Holocaust denial to the hate speech category and providing judges with latitude to levy higher penalties on individuals and groups convicted of racist delinquencies (not all were criminalized) (Bleich, 2001, 2003).

CONCLUSION

New Year 2017 brought with it headlines of murder and mayhem in the great American city of Chicago. Media outlets across the country reported that in 2016, Chicago's murder rate exceeded that of both New York and Los Angeles combined. Although sensationalized, the statistics represent an accurate depiction of how many citizens in the city of Chicago died at the hands of other citizens in one year. Not only is it true, but it actually warrants the quantity of discussion surrounding it. It is the quality and context of the discussion that is most disconcerting, although not surprising.

In 2010, Isabel Wilkerson's Pulitzer Prize winning work "The Warmth of Other Sons" was released. This book chronicled the lives of three families who moved from the Jim Crow South to the Northern and Mid-Western states seeking a life where they could be seen, heard and maybe even valued. Ms. Wilkerson's work was inspired by Richard Wright, who wrote:

> I was leaving the South to fling myself into the unknown ... I was taking a part of the South to transplant in alien soil, to see if it could grow differently, if it could drink of new and cool rains, bend in strange winds, respond to the warmth of other suns and, perhaps, to bloom. (Wright, 1998, p. 414)

The venerable Wright was describing his experience as he moved from Memphis to Chicago in 1927, at the age of 19. From 1915 through the early 1970s, millions of Black families moved to Chicago fueled by hope-filled spirits while simultaneously riddled with the traumas inflicted by their prior suns scathing burns. Journalist, talking heads, city bureaucrats and law enforcement officials implicate the crime and violence on gang members, weak gun use penalties and an emboldenment of criminals. To this list, they add an anti-police environment and even began to describe these "pockets of very bad people" responsible for the crime and violence. More than three generations after the first great migration and nearly two after the second, the progeny of these men and women in search of a better life are forced to watch their great and great-great grandchildren die in the streets. In 2016, there were over 4000 shooting victims and 462 homicides. What is different about the dreams of the 19-year-old Black man raised in the Jim Crow South from those of the 19-year-old Black man in contemporary Chicago? What is different about the Chicago that Richard Wright moved to almost a century ago?

It seems very easy for us to discuss crime and violence in a city like Chicago without addressing the etiology. We superficially blame the families. We simplify the identity of those whose pain might be operationalized in criminal behaviors simply as "criminals", easily forgetting the intergenerational deferment of dreams that plague their subconscious. Will we continue to refer to them as "pockets of very bad people"? Will we continue to seek out ways to increase the punishment when most psychological research has dismissed the efficacy of the "scared straight" punitive paradigm? What else are we doing for the city of Chicago and the residents there? Twelve of Chicago's murders in 2016 were a part of 27 shooting incidents just during the December holiday weekend. When pain runs so deep that the goal of the shooter is to ensure the loved ones of his foe bear witness to and absorb the resultant trauma, there is a problem that is significant and has gone long unaddressed.

Major cities around the world can continue using their strategic subject algorithms to identify repeat offenders of gun violence. They can work with neighboring counties and states to halt the influx of fire arms obtained under less restrictive guidelines. They can even increase objectives related to community-oriented policing models. These efforts, although good and necessary, fail to address the true underlying factors informing gang involvement, gang violence and shooting deaths in urban cities across the globe.

Some contend that the evidence points to a more deliberate and insidious plan to maintain the marginalization of poor people, particularly people of color who exist at the intersection of the poverty line. Most of the violence in Chicago is almost isolated in two major geographic areas, both of which are largely populated by people of color experiencing poverty. In addition to pain, these are communities demonstrating great resilience and strength, yet they are often described as those unwilling to "play by societies rules". As illustrated throughout this chapter, it appears that these communities have been violated—across many generations—by a system unwilling to facilitate equitable and inclusive societal rules.

To address this very problem, Brooklyn, NY, emergency physician Rob Gore established the Kings Against Violence Initiative (KAVI). In his Ted Talk *Healing Inner City Trauma*, he indicates that the Centers for Disease Control (CDC) confirms that the number one cause of death for Black men ages 15–34 is homicide. Dr. Gore goes on to discuss the limited psychosocial resources provided to survivors of inner city violence, particularly when compared to survivors of school or work place shootings where counselors are often dispatched without hesitation. KAVI approaches community violence from a public health framework addressing each system in which participants and their families exist. The program is built on a foundation that acknowledges etiological risk factors that contribute to the development of community violence. Restricted access to an affirming education, inadequate access to culturally empathic mental wellness programs and communities with severely limited resources and services must all be addressed when taking a holistic approach to violence intervention and prevention in urban communities across the world.

Without taking this entire contextual history into consideration, many are compelled to objectify Black men and boys as the post-emancipation historical record demonstrates through systems like debt peonage and convict leasing. This objectification—not unlike misogynistic objectification—dehumanizes the target. This dehumanization renders their responses to authentic pain and injustice pathological, churlish or innately hedonistic. This perspective is *not* aimed at absconding individuals from personal accountability and collective responsibility for actions in which they engaged. It *is* aimed at ensuring that a richer understanding is created to support a wider ecological framework for contemporary concerns that have historical roots.

References

American Psychiatric Association. (2013). *Diagnostic and Statistical Manual of Mental Disorders* (5th ed.). Washington, DC: Author.

Babu, S., & Banerjee, M. (2017). Understanding Epigenetics of Schizophrenia in the Backdrop of Its Antipsychotic Drug Therapy. *Epigenomics, 9*(5), 721–736.

Beach, S., Brody, G., Kit Lei, M., Simons, R., Philibert, R., Cutrona, C., et al. (2013). Impact of Child Sex Abuse on Adult Psychopathology: A Genetically and Epigenetically Informed Investigation. *Journal of Family Psychology, 27*(1), 3–11.

Bleich, E. (2001). *Race Policy in France.* Brookings. Retrieved from https://www.brookings.edu/articles/race-policy-in-france/

Bleich, E. (2003). *Race Politics in Britain and France: Ideas and Policymaking Since the 1960's.* Cambridge: Cambridge University Press.

Brave-Heart, M. Y. H. (2014). *Historical Trauma and Unresolved Grief: Implications for Clinical Research and Practice with Indigenous Peoples of the Americas.* Presentation. Retrieved February 21, 2018, from https://www.ihs.gov/telebehavioral/includes/themes/newihstheme/display_objects/documents/slides/education/historicaltrauma_100412.pdf

Bronfenbrenner, U. (1994). *Ecological Models of Human Development. International Encyclopedia of Education* (Vol. 3, 2nd ed.). Oxford: Elsevier. Reprinted in: Gauvin, M., & Cole, M. (Eds.), *Readings on the Development of Children* (2nd Ed., pp. 37–43, 1993). New York: Freeman.

Catterall, P. (1997). What (If Anything) Is Distinctive About Contemporary History? *Journal of Contemporary History, 32*(4), 441–452. Sage Publications.

Chial, H., & Craig, J. (2008). mtDNA and Mitochondrial Diseases. *Nature Education, 1*(1), 217.

Coyle, S. (2014). Intergenerational Trauma—Legacies of Loss. *Social Work Today, 14*(3), 18.

Dallaire, R. (2015). *Shake Hands with the Devil; The Failure of Humanity in Rwanda.* Toronto: Random House.

Diallo, R. (2018). *France Dangerous Move to Remove 'Race' From Its Constitution.* Washington Post. Retrieved from https://www.washingtonpost.com/news/global-opinions/wp/2018/07/13/frances-dangerous-move-to-remove-race-from-its-constitution/?noredirect=on&utm_term=.6aaf3dad6189

European Commission. (2017). *Diversity and Inclusion Charter.* Retrieved from https://ec.europa.eu/info/sites/info/files/diversity-inclusion-charter-2017-07-19-en.pdf

European Network Against Racism. Retrieved from https://www.enar-eu.org/About-us

Gabbidon, S., & Taylor, H. (2012). *Race and Crime: A Text/Reader.* Thousand Oaks, CA: Sage Publishing.

Gone, J. P. (2014). Reconsidering American Indian Historical Trauma: Lessons from an Early Gros Ventre War Narrative. *Transcultural Psychiatry, 51*(3), 387–406.

Hagengimana, A., Hinton, D., Bird, B., Pollack, M., & Pitman, R. K. (2003). Somatic Panic-Attack Equivalents in a Community Sample of Rwandan Widows Who Survived the 1994 Genocide. *Psychiatry Research, 117*(1), 1–9.

Hamza, M., Halayem, S., Bourgou, S., Daoud, M., Charfi, F., & Belhadi, A. (2017). Epigenetics and ADHD: Toward an Integrative Approach of the Disorder Pathogenesis. *Journal of Attention Disorders, 23*(7), 655–664.

Javaid, N., & Choi, S. (2017). Acetylation- and Methylation-Related Epigenetic Proteins in the Context of Their Targets. *Genes, 198*(8), 1–37.

Jost, J., & Kay, A. (2010). Social Justice: History, Theory, and Research. In S. T. Fiske, D. Gilbert, & G. Lindzey (Eds.), *Handbook of Social Psychology* (Vol. 2, 5th ed., pp. 1122–1165). Hoboken, NJ: Wiley.

Kellerman, N. (2008). Transmitted Holocaust Trauma: Curse or Legacy? The Aggravating and Mitigating Factors of Holocaust Transmission. *Israeli Journal of Psychiatric and Related Sciences, 45*(4), 263–270.

Kirmayer, L., Gone, J., & Moses, J. (2014). Rethinking Historical Trauma. *Transcultural Psychiatry, 51*(3), 299–319.

League for the Fifth International. *The Oppression of Black People in the USA Today*. Retrieved from http://www.fifthinternational.org/content/oppression-Black-people-usa-today

Leduc, S., & Frosch, J. (2013). *Black Public Figures Sound Alarm on 'Racist France'*. France 24. Retrieved from https://www.france24.com/en/20131106-france-racism-christiane-taubira-harry-roselmack-marine-le-pen-nicolassarkozy

Levingston, S. (2017). *Kennedy and King; The President, the Pastor, and the Battle over Civil Rights*. New York: Hachette Books.

Little, D. (2012). *Analytical Sociology and the Rest of Sociology*. Sociologica 1/2012. Societa editrice il Mulino Bologna. Retrieved from http://www.gemass.org/manzo/sites/default/files/2_little.pdf

Mamdani, M. (2002). *When Victims Become Killers: Colonialism, Nativism and the Genocide in Rwanda*. Princeton, NJ: Princeton University Press.

Moynihan, D. P. (1965). *The Negro Family: The Case for National Action*. Office of Policy Planning and Research. US Department of Labor. Retrieved from https://web.stanford.edu/~mrosenfe/Moynihan's%20The%20Negro%20Family.pdf

Papirblat, S. (2017). *Belgian Ice Cream Company Causes Uproar Over 'Racist' Chocolate Specialty*. Israel: Haaretz. Retrieved from http://www.fifthinternational.org/content/oppression-Black-people-usa-today

Penal Code Article 226-19. Retrieved from http://www.track.unodc.org/LegalLibrary/LegalResources/France/Laws/France%20Penal%20Code.pdf

Peroud, N., Rutembesa, E., Paoloni-Giacabino, A., Mutesa, L., Malafosse, A., & Karege, F. (2014). The Tutsi Genocide and Transgenerational Transmission of Maternal Stress: Epigenetics and Biology of the HPA Axis. *The World Journal of Biological Psychiatry, 15*(4), 334–345.

Rankin, J. (2018). *Is the EU Too White- and Brexit Likely to Make It Worse. MEPs and Staff Say*. The Guardian. Retrieved from https://www.theguardian.com/world/2018/aug/29/eu-is-too-white-brexit-likely-to-make-it-worse

Robinson, C. (2000). *Black Marxism: The Making of the Black Radical Tradition*. Chapel Hill, NC: University of North Carolina Press.

Rushton, J. P. (1997). *Race, Evolution, and Behavior: A Life History Perspective*. New Brunswick, NJ: Transaction Publishers.

Salas, A., Carrecedo, A., Richard, M., & Macaulay, V. (2005). Charting the Ancestry of African Americans. *American Journal of Human Genetics, 77*(4), 676–680.

Schroeder, H., Avila-Arcos, M., Malaspinas, A.-S., Poznik, G. D., Sandoval-Velasco, M., Carpenter, M. L., et al. (2015). Genome-Wide Ancestry of 17th-Century Enslaved Africans from the Caribbean. *PNAS, 112*(12), 3669–3673.

Silverman, R. C., & Lieberman, A. F. (1999). Negative Maternal Attributions, Projective Identification, and the Intergenerational Transmission of Violent Relational Patterns. *Psychoanalytic Dialogues, 9*(2), 161–186. https://doi.org/10.1080/10481889909539312

Sorrells, K. (2016). *Intercultural Communication: Globalization and Social Justice.* Thousand Oaks, CA: Sage Publications.

Stille, A. (2014). Can the French Talk About Race. *The New Yorker.* Retrieved from https://www.newyorker.com/news/news-desk/can-the-french-talk-about-race

Sussman, R. W. (2014). *The Myth of Race: The Troubling Persistence If an Unscientific Idea.* Boston: Harvard University Press.

The Local. (2015). *French Baker Forced to Remove 'Racist' Cake.* France. Retrieved from https://www.thelocal.fr/20150326/french-baker-forced-to-remove-racist-cakes

Udo-Akang, D. (2012). Theoretical Constructs, Concepts and Applications. *American International Journal of Contemporary Research, 2*(9), 89–97.

Vinovskis, M. (2005). *The Birth of Head Start: Preschool Educations Policies in the Kennedy and Johnson Administrations.* Chicago: University of Chicago Press.

Volcan, V. (2001). Transgenerational Transmissions and Chosen Traumas: An Aspect of Large-Group Identity. *Group Analysis, 34*(1), 79–98.

Weingarten, K. (2004). Witnessing the Effects of Political Violence in Families: Mechanisms of Intergenerational Transmission and Clinical Interventions. *Journal of Marital and Family Therapy, 30*(1), 1–40.

Wright, R. (1998). Black Boy. *Harper Perennial.*

Youssef, N., Lockwood, L., Su, S., Hao, G., & Rutten, B. (2018). The Effects of Trauma, With or Without PTSD, on the Transgenerational DNY Methylation Alterations in Human Offspring. *Journal of Brain Science, 8*(83), 1–7.

CHAPTER 5

Post-Traumatic Nooses: *Modern Eugenics and Mechanistic Media*

Social epidemiology illustrates the "effects of social-structural factors on states of health" and seeks societal characteristics that impact patterns of disease in order to understand etiology. This discipline might incorporate viewpoints from bio-psychosocial models, political and economic theories, the population perspective or significance theory (Honjo, 2004; Sotero, 2006). Social epidemiological approaches afford researchers and practitioners with the opportunity to truly see how systems create and sustain unique environments where outcomes can be both predicted and prevented.

Monsignor Theophilus Okere laments on the cruelty of the Transatlantic Slave Trade:

> Never before, nor since, has there been a commercial traffic in human beings of that magnitude, intensity or duration, involving such distances between four continents and lasting over four hundred years. Never did commerce ever involve so much contempt, so much cruelty and so much inhumanity tolerated or even supported by some of the highest moral minds and authorities, championed by the most Catholic countries of Europe. (Adiele, 2017 p. 2)

The decimation of slavery didn't occur over night. As early as the 1850s planters, investors, European slavers, British textile makers and French colonialists had reliable evidence that the institution was under a formidable threat of eradication. As the possibility of slavery's demise became more

© The Author(s) 2019   121
D. E. Grant Jr., *Black Men, Intergenerational Colonialism, and Behavioral Health*, https://doi.org/10.1007/978-3-030-21114-1_5

and more evident, the actors involved in the markets of this global economy began to panic. Protests, riots, legislation and wars have all been attributed to the dismantling of Black American enslavement. Given the synergies created by all these factors, it is unimaginable that stakeholders, slavery empathizers, plantation entrepreneurs or government officials in support of the institution never thought of risk management strategies as they faced the significant losses associated with the abolition of slavery. For those still unable to see the change on the horizon, even with all the signals, they were surely able to benefit from the two years between the signing of the Emancipation Proclamation in 1863, which provided figurative freedom for enslaved Blacks, and the thirteenth amendment to the American Constitution marking the nation's legally binding commitment to the promise of liberty for all. A detailed exploration of the perinatal events surrounding the birth of emancipation tells a story of tactical foresight and deliberate planning. Practice and policy liter the historical record demonstrating a very strategic and thoughtful method by which the benefits of a sun-setting free plantation labor force would be maintained to support the global economy it had just built. Stakeholders across the globe were running multi-million dollar empires, and the likelihood of "being caught off guard" by this change without a plan is preposterous.

Business continuity and continuity of operations planning are similar risk management strategies used to create resiliency tools for industries and organizations to enlist in the face of threats to business functions. The abolition of slavery in America and the global economic webs created by its proliferation housed many elements. When interrupted, these interconnected features had the capacity to topple an entire global economic industrial infrastructure. International trade relations, labor force costs, land procurement, markets for surplus goods, natural resource acquisition and continued cultural imperialism were all under severe threat in the face of this changing ecosystem. An efficient business continuity plan would include specific steps to take when an event foreshadows the loss of functionality, sustainability or viability of a particular business process. The Transatlantic Slave Trade and the sustained systematic enslavement of Black people represented the most significant business processes of the global economy at the time. It supported the development of international trade relationships, provided a cost-free labor force, opened amiable access to global markets, built a knowledge base for natural resource stripping and trained practitioners of cultural and physical genocide. Global stakeholders would in fact employ several successful risk management strategies to ensure the continuity of business operations in the face of these significant risks.

Eugenics, convict leasing and debt peonage, African colonization, psychological testing, government experimentation and the institutionalization of racism are all examples of strategies used in the business continuity model of global economic stakeholders facing colossal landscape changes. Many individuals, businesses and groups benefitted from the random cross-pollination of ideas and experiences, while others deliberately convened to develop these strategies. Steps included in the life cycles of most successful business continuity models begin with a solution design which is followed by its implementation. Once implemented, design components are tested for fit and eventually accepted into the system. To ensure that the model works, each component must be maintained and continuously analyzed in the case that time demonstrates additional re-adjustments. The approaches employed to implement and test strategies aimed at the maintenance of slavery provide a body of evidence that led to their acceptance as preferable tactics to both preserve the status quo and expand spheres of exploitative influence. The chosen practices would evolve with the changing world into contemporary recapitulations of themselves aimed to maintain the critical outcomes associated with their original iterations.

In addition to the explicit modernization of historic tools of oppression, those in power added additional tactics to serve as binding agents to ensure long-term operational continuity. The arbitrary and unwarranted colonization of Africa followed by the haphazard decolonization effectively created a narrative of destabilization and mistrust resulting in a set of acrimonious relationships between men and women of African descent across the diaspora, ensuring divisions to increase global conquerability. The institutionalization of racism and colorism thrives daily in the lives of men of African descent as they are barred from employment opportunities, snubbed for promotions, denied access to academic enrichment, vilified across media outlets, deprived of professional mentorship, victimized by scientific racism and systematically removed from their families and communities by deliberately placed infrastructural fractures.

The American Civil War, the Emancipation Proclamation and the 13th Amendment to the American constitution dismantled the economic system that had endured untethered for over three centuries. The consequences were disastrous for businesses, and they needed a very strategic plan to avoid a total demise of their wealth and investments. The free labor provided by enslaved Blacks would have to be replaced somehow, if not at the same free rate, something close to nothing was required to maintain the pre-emancipation profit margins. The American Civil War officially ended in 1865, and cotton began to flow slowly back into Britain as the Cotton Famine came to an end. As a result of specific strategies, processing plants in Manchester and Lancashire reopened and many people were able to regain full employment with confidence. The average British man would bounce back and continue to reap the benefits of the post-cotton famine industrialization, marking the advent of the British working class. This would not be the case with the Black American man who would be emancipated into an ecology deliberately structured to ensure the reestablishment of his bondage.

Black people were deprived of the freedom granted to them by the American government and its Constitution. It was clear the American Civil War had not diminished the world's need for cotton production. The world had become accustomed to the convenience of cotton and cotton-based textiles. As a result, newly freed people were often forced to stay in the south and work abandoned cotton plantations. They were not allowed to leave said plantation without a pass and were paid around $10 per month (Blackmon, 2008). Penalties for missing work were swift and severe. Cotton producers had utilized credit lines from the banking industries that they were now unable to repay, particularly if they had the new expense of paid labor. In most cases, the original terms of loans and structure of plantation taxation were made under favorable cotton prices that no longer existed. It was a challenging time in America. The livelihood of millions was directly linked to the global costs of cotton. As the debts of the planters increased so did the need for free Black labor and the malevolent methods to procure this labor (Blackmon, 2008).

A Despotic Trifecta: Sharecroppers, Debt Peons, Leased Convicts

The thirteenth amendment to the American Constitution states that "Neither slavery nor involuntary servitude, except as a punishment for crime whereof the party shall have been duly convicted, shall exist within the United States, or any place subject to their jurisdiction" (US Const. amend. XIII, sec. 1). The amendment clearly and decisively criminalizes the practice of slavery under any name in the USA or any of its protectorates. Prominently imbedded in this amendment is the unambiguously strategic exception to the nations' right to enslave a portion of its citizenry. Prior to 1865 in the USA, enslavement was a mandated condition predicated upon race, ethnic origin and the status of one's birth mother. As of January 1866, according to the 13th Amendment to the US Constitution, slavery was solely defined as a "punishment for crime" after one has been convicted. During the exact same moment in American history, eligibility for enslavement came to require a criminal conviction, the Southern states passed the Vagrancy Act of 1866 which was one part of a larger group of laws and regulations that strategically criminalized the formerly enslaved.

America would soon reclaim its crown as the number one producer and exporter of cotton in the world. By 1880, they were not only producing more cotton than they had in 1860, they had also grown cotton manufacturing plants in numbers never before seen in the country (Beckert, 2014). How is it possible that a business built upon the foundation of slave labor is able to not only sustain itself, but grow and thrive when the free-labor market upon which it was built is no longer at its disposal? The simple answer is a set of business continuity interventions that would secure free to low cost labor for small plantations and farms, large plantations and the Southern states whose infrastructure was severely damaged during the Civil War. Networks of small abandoned farms and plantations relied upon systems of sharecropping and debt peonage to reestablish their business. Many large unmanned plantations once imprisoned 200 plus enslaved people. Their scope of need could not be sufficiently met with the sharecropping model so they relied upon convict leasing programs. State governments and southern manufacturers also relied on convict leasing programs to repair roads, railroads and buildings severely compromised and rendered inaccessible by the war. The need for cheap labor was pronounced. How would this picture-perfect strategy be employed to ensure future prosperity given this critical change in the landscape (Blackmon, 2008).

As in most cases, it is hard to determine the intent of historic actions and decisions. What is not debatable is the fact that the most cost-effective labor plan in the American South had ended. In today's world, changes in laws and regulations that impact the labor force or availability of workers occur regularly. Most responsible business owners, c-suite executives and trustee boards have in place business continuity plans in the case internal or external factors lead to significant changes in their discipline or areas of responsibility. There is sufficient evidence (empirical and anecdotal) to conclude that these programs—share cropping, convict leasing and debt peonage—were central to the southern post-bellum guarantee for ongoing operations. New state constitutions ended the federal statutes that supported access for newly emancipated Blacks. Plessey v Ferguson provided federal support for institutionalized legal segregation and state laws took funding from Black schools, limited their access to goods and services and increased brutality against them (Franklin & Moss, 1988). The specific and measurable deliverable in this successful section of the business continuity plan was the re-enslavement of Black American men for the maintenance of both a proximate antebellum profit margin in the new plantation economy and a cut-rate labor force to support "reconstruction" of the American south.

In 1865, the *Macon Telegraph* of Georgia printed: "the great question now before our people is how to appropriate all the African labor of the country" (Beckert, 2014). Sentiments from the international community fell across the entire continuum of responses to the current conditions of America. In *The Cotton Supply of the United States of America*, an English businessman states: "Cotton can only be cultivated extensively in the Southern States by negro labour, and negro labour can only be controlled under the semi-patriarchal system called slavery" (Beckert, 2014). Whether enslaved or not, many of the global economic stakeholders rallied for the continued involvement of Black men and women in the cultivation of cotton. The entire system across the world worked heedfully to ensure that Southern Black Americans were thrust back into the condition of involuntary servitude similar to what they had experienced across ten generations. Although the plans of these multi-disciplinary teams—planters, politicians, jailers, industry—were multi-layered, there were three strategies that supported the largest catchment for the re-enslavement of Blacks in the former Confederate States of America. Slavery was rebranded, and the new southern trinity of bondage was comprised of the sharecropper, the convict and the debt peon. This trifecta would force Blacks back into the fields against their will for several more decades until they, like the institution of chattel slavery, were forced to evolve into systems of oppression and repression palatable for contemporary despots.

Sharecropping was a system of agricultural work that existed in Europe and colonial Africa before becoming a common arrangement among emancipated Blacks in the North American South during Reconstruction. In and of itself, sharecropping as a construct is not exploitative. Two-thirds of all sharecroppers were poor Southern Whites, and although they were all at the bottom of the social and economic American ladders, the Black sharecroppers experienced the brunt of the discriminatory practices. There are global examples, both historic and contemporary, where share-cropping, tenant farming and share-farming have all resulted in benefits for the land owner and the tenant renting land to farm upon. In most US cases, the sharecropper would purchase materials like animals, tools, seeds and fertilizer from the landowners on credit in order to grow their crops. Although there were sharecroppers of all races in the southern United States, narrative, anecdotal and empirical data of records from the time demonstrate that Black sharecroppers were consistently and frequently taken advantage of and further disenfranchised (Blackmon, 2008; Franklin & Moss, 1988).

As a result of the unfair practices of land owners, high interest rates and unpredictable harvests, sharecroppers were also often forced to procure other survival goods on credit from the land owners and local merchants like clothing and medical care costs. Henry Blanks was born enslaved in 1863, and was a small boy when he and his family were freed. His family worked as sharecroppers for a while after the American Civil War, and in his narrative, he shares the injustices associated with the agricultural system of sharecropping.

> When we worked on shares, we couldn't make nothing, just overalls and something to eat. Half went to the other man and you would destroy your half if you weren't careful. A man that didn't know how to count would always lose. He might lose anyhow. They didn't give no itemized statement. No, you just had to take their word. They never give you no details. They just say you owe so much. No matter how good accounting you kept, you had to go by their account and now, Brother, I'm tellin' you the truth about this. It's been that way for a long time … You could git anything you wanted as long as you worked. If you didn't make no money, that's all right; they would advance you more. But you better not leave him … They'd keep you in debt. They were sharp. Christmas come, you could take up twenty dollar, in somethin' to eat and much as you wanted in whiskey. You could buy a gallon of whiskey. Anything that kept you a slave because he was always right and you were always wrong … If there was an argument, he would get mad and there would be a shooting. (Arkansas Federal Writers Project)

Sharecropping contracts took many different forms. Many of the contracts evolved into land and crop-sharing arrangements where Black workers rented plots of land or were given plots to tend for a percentage of the land's yield. Land owners gained more control and began to implement very clear repressive instruments to disenfranchise Black workers and their progeny. For many Black families, sharecropping quickly became a new form of slavery.

In Covington Georgia, John S. Williams and his overseer, Clyde Manning, were facing murder charges for killing 11 Black men who had been held on his land illegally under the system of peonage. Peonage also known as debt-slavery was the practice of maintaining a person's indebtedness to control their labor. Outlawed by Congress in 1867, peonage is currently defined by federal statute 42 USCS § 1994 as "a condition of enforced servitude by which the servitor is compelled to labor against his will in liquidation of some debt or obligation, either real or pretend". A multitude of violations to this outlawed practice continued to come to the attention of local authorities and federal courts for decades after the Civil War. Records of court testimony demonstrate both how widespread this practice was and how far into the twentieth century the practice lasted.

As late as the early twentieth century, men like Williams had a practice of finding jailed Black men, paying their fines and taking them to their plantations to work off their debt (Daniel, 1972). Most of these planters never intended to free the men and had developed a system that to the naked eye was operationally identical to slavery, overseer and all. On Williams' plantations specifically, there were no records of him and his sons ever having released any of these men, nor were there records of wage rates or timelines by which the fines—many of them small—would ever be paid off. In Fall of 1920, two men were able to independently escape their illegal bondage on the Williams plantation. Both James Strickland and Gus Chapman fled to Atlanta where they disclosed their imprisonment and the atrocities that Williams and his sons engaged in to the Justice Department. Legal chattel slavery had ended nearly 60 years prior to their escape (Blackmon, 2008; Daniel, 1972).

Strickland and Chapman sparked an investigation leading federal investigators to rural Georgia to begin examining the allegations of the men. Following the investigators' first visit, Williams and Manning would have brutally murdered 11 people in an attempt to get rid of the evidence of twentieth-century slavery. During the trial, federal agent A.J. Wismer indicated that the Black people he interviewed on Williams' plantation "... were afraid to tell anything for fear they would tell the wrong things and would get into trouble and be punished there on the plantation" (Daniel, 1972, p. 123). The testimony in the trial, particularly that of Manning, described truly the horrendous murders. In his description, he was forced to commit the murders. "It was against my will to do it, but it was against my power not to do it and live" (Daniel, 1972, p. 130). In his testimony, he described each murder with great detail. He described the specific people they murdered, the way in which they were murdered and what his role was in this rampage. Some were hanged and some were drowned while others were beaten to death.

In 1921, both Williams and Manning were found guilty of first-degree murder and sentenced to life in prison. Williams was the first White man indicted for murdering a Black man since 1877, and it wouldn't happen again until 1966. Manning's attorneys would successfully appeal his case due to an omission regarding the intentionality and malice required for first-degree charges. During his second trial, Black men and women who had lived through the terrors of the Williams plantation described conditions that truly showed the insidiousness of peonage. Many of these men and women had spent their entire adult lives on this plantation, miles away from people who would act to stop the practice. Williams was killed in prison. Manning would die on a chain gang during the life sentence that resulted from his second trial. Williams' sons who had fled to Florida prior to the investigation were never charged (Blackmon, 2008; Daniel, 1972).

Much of the country was outraged at the notion that a practice such as peonage could prevail so far into the twentieth century. There were many cases beyond that of the Williams plantation. Governor Hugh M. Dorsey published a pamphlet entitled, "The Negro in Georgia" (Pitts, 2005) in 1922 which compiled the occurrences of lynching, peonage and cruelty, exposing the horrors of rural Georgia. For contextual purposes, while Marcus Garvey was launching the United Negro Improvement Association and Black fraternity and sorority chapters were being chartered on college campuses across the nation, rural Blacks were still being held as slaves on southern plantations as though it were the 1820s and not the 1920s.

Federal investigations in places like Texas, Georgia and Alabama placed violators of the peonage laws under close surveillance. Grand juries in Alabama began to issue indictments, opening their eyes to the actual scope of peonage. The National Archives hold letters and testimonies from family members requesting the freedom of their loved ones who were being held involuntarily by former slave owners in the south. These were planters who were well aware that emancipation had already been granted. In many of these letters, addressed directly to President Roosevelt, Blacks pleaded for assistance, prayed for support and hoped for the freedom of their loved ones.

The US Justice Department, the NAACP, the US Attorney's Office and other allies spoke against the atrocities of peonage. Circular 3591 submitted in December of 1941 identified an aggressive prosecutorial framework for any form if involuntary servitude, not just peonage. This was a part of Roosevelt's efforts to support increased rights for Black citizens. Eighty thousand people were forced into involuntary servitude during the decades after emancipation (Blackmon, 2008; Franklin & Moss, 1988).

Using prisoners and those convicted of crimes for the purposes of intense free labor was neither new nor unusual. Penal colonies, prison farms, debtor's colonies and indentured servitude were all ways in which municipal governments capitalized upon the labor capacities of individuals convicted of crimes. England, France and Russia utilized this technique for centuries throughout history to support the growth of their overseas investments. The British used North America as a penal colony where an estimated 50,000 British prisoners were shipped over and auctioned off to plantation owners as indentured servants, representing almost one-fourth of the English who emigrated from their country of origin. Convicts were used to build the Royal Naval Dockyard in Bermuda during the Second Boer War. These colonies persisted into the twentieth century in places like the Portuguese penal colony of Tarrafal in the Cape Verde Islands established in 1936. Convict Leasing Programs have their American origins in the south and grew exponentially after the liberation of the West Indian, Afro-Latinx and African American people. Southern states leased prisoners to municipal governments, railroad companies, coal mines and former slave plantations to grow cotton, tobacco and sugar. They were subject to unforgivingly harsh and deadly conditions without compensation (Blackmon, 2008).

In 2018, the bodies of almost 100 Black prison laborers and enslaved people were unearthed at a school construction site in Sugar Land, Texas. Testing of the remains indicated that the individuals ranged in ages from 14 to over 60 years old at their time of death. The remains showed signs of malnutrition and stress with skeletal markers evidencing participation in highly laborious activities. Bio-archaeologist Dr. Catrina Banks-Whitley, in her 2018 interview with ABC News (KTRK), stated "When you do activity over and over and over again, and you're doing heavy labor, it will actually stress the attachments where the muscles are attached to the bone. It will actually change the shape of the bone". Buried along with the bodies were chains, shackles, nails and manacles used to keep the convicts from fleeing and to remind them that they remained enslaved under this new American strategy. Were these individuals kept in bondage after the country ended its chapter as participants in the trade of enslaved people? Were they enslaved, freed and then imprisoned to return to their former life in bondage? We may never have the answers to those questions, but the one thing we can be sure of are the economic benefits that the plantation economy provided to the world, specifically sparking the British Industrial Revolution and catalyzing Global Capitalism. This economic model thrived upon a foundation of a legal institution of free and perpetual slave labor … until it didn't. Researchers believe that the cemetery was used from 1878 through 1910 (CBS News, 2018).

Convict leasing programs, supported by the Southern states, began in the middle of the nineteenth century. Prior to the Civil War, these organizations were able to lease both convicts and enslaved people to work the plantations, the mills, the mines and the railroads. The practice of leasing out prisoners for labor to these same entities became far more prevalent after the American Civil War, particularly since there were no more "slaves" to lease. Records indicate that Alabama, Texas, Arkansas, Mississippi, Florida, the Carolinas and other southern states participated in the utilization of incarcerated Blacks for further involuntary servitude while capitalizing on the practice (Blackmon, 2008).

In *Slavery by Another Name* (Blackmon, 2008), the author describes the convict leasing system as:

> … a form of bondage distinctly different from that of the antebellum South in that for most men, and relatively few women drawn in, this slavery did not last a lifetime and did not automatically extend from one generation to the next. But it was nonetheless slavery—a system in which armies of free men, guilty of no crimes and entitled by law to freedom, were compelled to labor without compensation, were repeatedly bought and sold, and were forced to do the bidding of White masters through the regular application of extraordinary physical coercion. (Blackmon, 2008, p. 4)

Free Black men and poor Whites were now on constitutional equal footing due to the adoption of the 13th Amendment. This presented a severe threat to White men and women, particularly as it manifested itself in Black men voting and serving as government officials all while the creation of schools for their children commenced. Even though they were now free, they were subject to municipal laws that had not existed in America's past, novel legislation for a newly reconstructed South. Offenses like spitting, walking aside a railroad track, loitering, pan handling or just existing in post-enslavement insolvency constituted imprisonment and hard labor.

The end of American slavery led to the liberation of over 3 million people in the USA. The vast majority of those recently freed were unable to read or write, had never lived independently and had just been released from a condition riddled with unaddressed traumas that were horrifically complex. The state of Mississippi implemented the very first American Black Codes in 1865. This comprehensive set of practices and laws that applied explicitly to Black people was in many ways simply a remix of the slave codes to account for the federal emancipation of this group. Some of these codes demanded that Black workers enter into labor contracts with White farmers at the start of each year or risk being arrested. South Carolina followed adoption and actually quantified one-eighth as the threshold of blackness that would render one subject to the enforcements of these codes. Other states passed laws that bound Black workers to the plantation where they worked by requiring them to procure discharge papers before being able to be legally hired by any other employer (Blackmon, 2008; Franklin & Moss, 1988).

The act of vagrancy—as defined in the Vagrancy Act of 1866—is committed when one appears to be unemployed or homeless. Upon emancipation, most Blacks had no permanent residence as they searched for work and loved ones who were ripped from their hearts during their enslavement. This would effectively criminalize most every newly emancipated Black man and woman. As a result, every set of Southern Black Codes were girded with the act of vagrancy as a cornerstone component of each state's individual codes. This was used to oblige freedmen to become signatories in their own re-enslavement. White Americans were not subject to any of these rules of law. Blacks, often sentenced to death for things like arson, rebellion and assaulting a White woman, were now also being arrested for minor offenses that were not crimes for those with less than 12.5% Black blood running through their veins (Baptiste, 2015; Blackmon, 2008; Franklin & Moss, 1988). In order to effectively utilize convicts for leasing, the state institutions had to have enough prisoners to meet the southern demand. Only 10% of the people arrested during Reconstruction were White. The highest lease rates paid were for the strongest men and those with the longest sentences. In fall when it was time to harvest cotton, arrests would increase substantially. More than two-thirds of the arrests during this time were for burglary and larceny (Blackmon, 2008).

John Turner Milner, born in Alabama in 1826, was an experienced Southern businessman, engineer and politician who gained wealth in coal, gold and railroads. He is noted throughout history as a major catalyzing actor in the convict leasing programs of Alabama. In 1864 during their first year leasing convicts to state governments, private businesses and plantation owners, the state of Alabama earned $14,000 ($426,000 in 2019 dollars). Twenty-six years later, in 1890, they had earned $164,000 ($4.6 million in 2019 dollars) representing more than a 1000% increase in yield. Some of the first railroads in Alabama were completed by convicts leased to the state and private entities responsible for the lines. Other states joined Alabama in this leasing program and business grew exponentially (Milner, 1890).

In 1890, Milner's pamphlet, *White Men of Alabama Stand Together*, was published. In it, he consistently describes his lack of prejudice and even unambiguously supports the emancipation of enslaved Africans. In a very oxymoronic way, he would also berate them, aggregating pseudo-science and false-hearted evidence to reinforce a narrative of barbarianism, laziness and a people devoid of any ability to self-govern. He makes observations of several colonies who saw a decline in production of agricultural goods after emancipation, describes the lack of will and desire in the newly freed Blacks as the reason the once profitable plantation crops had reverted to mere "bush". He further demonstrates how a drop in per capita production for individual Blacks when compared to pre-emancipation rates caused the economic demise of several Caribbean and West Indian nations. Through an exploration of African manumissions across European colonies, he suggests, that when left to their own free will, emancipated Blacks would certainly devolve, stating: "Their descendants have all been emancipated now, some for nearly 100 years, and some for hardly one. They have ... everywhere retrograded and gone back to barbarism" (Milner, 1890, p. 3).

Prior to emancipation, thousands of enslaved people were used across a variety of southern industries. Alabama coal mines from the 1830s through the Civil War relied upon enslaved men who were leased from plantation owners. Coal and steel mines in Alabama, Georgia and Tennessee were also largely run by enslaved men. Railroad companies leased thousands of enslaved people to lay the foundation for the first interstate systems of transportation and commerce. It is estimated that the railroad companies controlled 20,000 enslaved Blacks at the start of the American Civil War (Blackmon, 2008). The short window of time that passed before a plan had been implemented to maintain this labor force across industries was striking. There are records of cotton plantation contracts for newly freed men as early as 1866, the year following the 13th Amendments inclusion into the US Constitution. This contractual relationship between the landowner and the freedman often indicated that they work from sunrise to sunset, be available for additional activities after sunset and commit to tending the plantation on Sundays (Beckert, 2014).

Milner also owned coal mines where he had a penchant for using prisoners for work. The convicts mined coal under brutal conditions, very similar to that of their enslaved parents. The overseers of the convicts in the coal mines and on the plantations were often previous slave owners. Convict miners cost significantly less than the paid miners. They could be rented for as little as $9.00 per month, creating a major difference in financial investment between the convicts and the enslaved. This also very often resulted in a different paradigm of treatment for the convicts when compared to the enslaved (Blackmon, 2008).

Purchasing people for enslavement was a significant fiduciary venture. Due to the financial investment of the purchased human being and their capacity to birth or impregnate, enslaved people would be beaten, maimed and brutalized within inches of death but often sparred from its liberating finality. The investment made in a leased convict was miniscule, and the incarcerated pool of convicts to lease was growing exponentially due to a successful implementation of a model business continuity plan. The brutality of this new iteration of enslavement became, by some accounts, even more heartless than its predecessor. Plantation owners, government officials, overseers, miners and other entrepreneurs had little incentive to treat these convicts with any humanity. During enslavement, if an enslaved man or woman was killed, that planter was out of a great deal of money. The only way to replace this loss was to replace the murdered slave with a new one. When the convicts were beaten to the cusp of death, the motivation to engage in any self-control is minimized due to the lack of financial risk. If this prisoner were to die, the plantation owner would just go and lease more prisoners. The death rates of convict leases were high, as much as 30–40%. Death rates for leased convicts from Alabama in 1866 and 1867 was 20%. By 1870, nearly 45% of these men would be murdered while being leased out by the state of Alabama (Blackmon, 2008).

In 1877—as Reconstruction was coming to an end—every state that once made up the former Confederate States of America, with the exception of Virginia, was engaged in the practice of leasing Black prisoners to agents of commerce, government and infrastructure industry (Blackmon,

2008). In 1886, there were 15,000 prisoners working as leased convicts; on average, the number would grow by 1000 each year—almost 20 new prisoners leased every week—over the next four years. By 1890, there were 19,000 convicts being leased across the American south, and the overwhelmingly vast majority of them were Black men (Baptiste, 2015; Blackmon, 2008). By the end of the nineteenth century, Black codes and vagrancy laws rendered Blacks severely over-represented in the US prison population. This would mark the birth of new narratives that resulted in an array of intuitive associations between freed Blacks and criminality. Now that these men could no longer be "slaves", they would now be subject to innate membership in a new under-class, that of convict. Today, this narrative continues to haunt Black men and boys across the world, rendering them subject to disproportionate surveillance, harassment by security officers, murders by law enforcement, skepticism by banking institution management and discrimination by café employees.

Convict contracts made it such that the families who leased the prisoners were able to beat them, hunt them and even murder them. Many of the wealthy farmers of the south had their own "justice of the peace", providing them with the opportunity to secure convictions for men to effectively re-enslave them within the eye of the law. The federal government fought against Black Codes and continued support for freedmen until the end of the1870s when the last Union soldiers left the former Confederate. By this time, many vigilante groups had been incubating in the southern country sides where the Ku Klux Klan began their reign of terror. Once the south was left to its own devices, the Black Codes evolved into Jim Crow and continued to saturate the southern life of Black men and their families with the poisons of what they believed had been their unrepeatable pasts (Blackmon, 2008).

Much of our American criminal justice system was firmly established while racism and segregation ruled the South. During this time, the rules that governed Blacks began as the slave codes, evolved into Black Codes and grew into Jim Crow. It is not a surprise that we continue to see Black men disproportionately punished, unscrupulously arrested, randomly accosted and brutally murdered for rules, practices and policies that appear to only apply to them, particularly when penance is attached. We continue to see an array of Black males punished for code violations that are either not applied to or attended to when perpetrated by their White male counterparts.

MODERN-DAY CONTINUITY

Contemporary infrastructure resulting from the aforementioned global business continuity strategies has been maintained through a series of procedural evolutions and creative nomenclature alterations. The application of a comparative lens unearths some uncanny similarities between activities used to maintain the subjugation of Blacks immediately following nineteenth-century emancipation and efforts that support those similar goals across the past two centuries. These tools and tactics are present and prevalent in the USA, the UK, Canada and France.

Convict leasing, relied upon heavily after emancipation, might be viewed as maintained contemporarily in the deficits-based reintegration programs for those leaving prison or jail, the unbalanced surveillance and search policies of urban centers, disparate adjudication practices, bail and bond structures, expungement policies and an unjustifiably disproportionate rate of over-incarceration. Debt peonage, another tool birthed by slavery's death, lives today as prohibitive educational costs, predatory pay day loan practices and the restriction of specific civil rights following incarceration.

In 2018 alone, the USA saw a teen arrested at Wolfchase Galleria Mall in Memphis for violating the malls dress code (Kenney, 2018), an Arizona teen handcuffed and arrested for an unclear dress code violation at Apache Junction High School and referred to the Pinal County Juvenile Court System (Hamlin, 2018), a Milwaukee Bucks basketball player arrested and shot with a stun gun by officers over a parking violation (Domonoske & Brown, 2018) and two men arrested for awaiting a colleague's arrival at a Philadelphia coffee shop (Held, 2018). These represent a miniscule set of experiences that Black men and boys have as they are over surveilled, disproportionately punished and consistently given the harshest punishments available for infractions which others receive nominal reprimands. This contemporary existence is not unique to America.

In a report entitled: *The Colour of Injustice: Race, Drugs and Law Enforcement in England and Wales Today*, researchers confirmed that Blacks in the UK were 8.7 times more likely to be stopped and searched for drugs under their "stop and search" powers and 7.9 times more likely (under the same practice) to be stopped for other offenses (Shiner, Carre, Delsol, & Eastwood, 2018). Although the detection rates from the stop and search tactics used in the UK are similar for all ethnic groups, arrests in the UK—like most Euronormative countries—are disproportionately

Black. During the 2016–2017 recording period, it was reported that there were 779,660 arrests in England and Wales. For Whites in this region, there were only 12 arrests per 1000 residents, while for Blacks, there were 30 per every 1000, showcasing a Black arrest rate almost three times that of their White counterparts. When this data is disaggregated around gender, the story gets exponentially worse. This same report demonstrates that 71 Black men are arrested per 1000 Black male residents. Across a 10-year period from 2006–2007 through 2016–2017, the overall number of arrests in England and Wales dropped by a little over 50%, the decrease for its Black arrests was just 32%. The highest arrest rates for Blacks in the UK were found in the Police Force Areas of Dorset, Cumbria, Cheshire, Avon & Somerset and Cleveland (Police Powers and Procedure England and Wales Statistics, 2018).

A similar study, *Profiling Minorities: A Study of Stop-and-Search Practices in Paris*, published by the Open Society Institute in 2009 confirmed that police stops and identity checks in Paris are "principally based on the appearance of the person stopped, rather than on their behaviors or actions" (Open Society Justice Initiative, 2009, p. 10). The study examined 500 police stops across five locations surrounding the Gare du Nord and Chaelet-Les Halles rail stations in central Paris from October 2007 through May 2008. Overall, Black residents were six times more likely than Whites to be stopped. The disproportionality ceiling across sites in this study demonstrated that Blacks in some areas were actually more than 11 times more likely to be stopped by police. The appearance criteria used were found to include not just phenotypic characteristics like skin color but style of clothes worn as well. Although only 10% of those of age to have been stopped by the police were dressed in clothing typically associated with the French youth culture, 47% of those stopped were described as a part of this group with styles described as "hip-hop", "tecktonic" or "punk". The study concluded that police consider both belonging to an ethnic minority group and wearing youth clothing to be closely tied to a propensity to commit crimes or infractions (Open Society Justice Initiative, 2009).

The *Report of the Commission on Systemic Racism in the Ontario Criminal Justice System* from 1995 demonstrated huge disparities in the ways that Blacks were treated and engaged throughout the province. One of the most striking statistics across the six-year period from 1986–1987 to 1992–1993 was that the Black prison population in Ontario grew by 204% juxtaposed to a 23% increase among Whites in Ontario (Commission on Systemic Racism in the Ontario Criminal Justice System, 1995). In 2017, the *Racial Profiling and Human Rights* was published by the Ontario Human Rights Commissioner and indicated that Black people are not only over-represented throughout the criminal justice system when compared to their White counterparts, but that they are also more likely to be: stopped, arrested and kept in jail. Although Canadian police have not historically collected data on the race of people detained or searched, data from Toronto's Police Service's Criminal Information System (CIPS) demonstrates that Black residents of Toronto were over-represented across many charge categories including driving and traffic charges, drug possessions and prostitution (Ontario Human Rights Commission, 2017).

In *The Presumption of Guilt*, Charles Ogletree describes several categories for which Black men are subject to undue risks for potential injustice and racial injury by law enforcement, peers, subordinates, superiors, service providers, customers and even children. Dr. Ogletree identifies the following general constructs as risk categories: Driving while Black, mistaken criminal accusation by law enforcement absent evidence, public suspicion of criminal behavior in neutral or ambiguous circumstances, stimulated unwarranted and unprompted fear in innocuous scenarios, presumption of servitude when a guest or host, over-surveillance and profiling by police, and disproportionate scrutiny of credentials (Ogletree, 2010).

For many people, these infractions either never happen or happen so infrequently that there is no impetus to identify a pattern, because there isn't one. For others, the frequency with which exposure occurs warrants a search for the responsible persons and/or systems. Every Black man in every Euronormative nation has experienced at least one race-related injury and remains in moment to moment danger of further confrontations. At times, these assaults fly so far below the radar of consciousness that they go unnoticed, not to be confused with innocuous. Dr. Ogletree uses the first-hand accounts of Black men as primary sources to evidence a deliberate pattern of malevolent engagement. From Justice Thurgood Marshall and former Attorney General Eric Holder to film director Douglas McHenry and radio host Warren Ballentine, these Black men of means join the ranks of middle-class Black men and those experiencing poverty in a universal experience.

There are times when these experiences among wealthy Black men mirror those of Black men living in poverty. Although each group and all those in between might be disproportionately targeted because of their race, it is important to note that more often than not socio-economic status mediates outcomes using status-based protective factors. Status-based protective factors are those ecological elements that afford privileged members of a sub-group opportunities to minimize impact and catalyze recovery when confronted with racial injuries across the continuum. Although supportive of resilience, these protective factors don't prevent racially injurious events from occurring as evidenced by on-going narratives from Black men representing most every life domain and geographic sphere dominated by standards and norms grounded in a White Eurocentric cultural tradition. Some of these factors include financial resource availability, access to superior legal counsel, mental bandwidth, multi-disciplinary healthcare and insurance, family and community support, education and secure housing.

Eugenics Then and Now

The people of ancient Egypt led lives dedicated to culture, art and expression. They enjoyed sports like wrestling and gymnastics. Some attended bullfighting matches and ball games, while others enjoyed orchestras and produced stage plays. Athenians consistently engaged in cultural activities like concerts and poetry readings. Their children played with dolls and kites while they enjoyed sports and art. This all occurred during a time when prosperity (for many) extended far and wide. The cotton industry created a British working/middle class with cognitive and emotional bandwidths to support leisure activities in a scope broader than what had existed in past generations. Evidence from the 1830s through the 1900s supports the new spaces in which the British existed, they were moving into another stage of national development. For Britain, this time was marked by the development of community parks, theaters, movie halls and country clubs. They hosted the first international cricket and football (soccer) matches and invented lawn tennis.

Leading up to this time of recreation and reflection, during the middle of the eighteenth century, central England had experienced a distinctive regional enlightenment in the middle of the broader European Age of Enlightenment. The Midlands Enlightenment, as it was known, became a scientific, economic, political, cultural and legal movement fueled by the exponential British industrial and economic growth of the time. The Lunar Society, an exclusive dinner discussion club for elite British intellectuals, English dissenters and scientists who met between 1765 and 1813, was central to this movement. Members met in and around Birmingham where their disciplines cross-pollinated to birth some of the most inventive and lucrative models of innovation. Their membership overtime included an interdisciplinary mix of thinkers and movers like industrialist Mathew Boulton, engineer James Watt and scientist Joseph Priestley.

The Midlands Enlightenment in general and the Lunar Society specifically created a space where the scientific revolution was able to merge with the industrial revolution. This link resulted in a unique synergistic regional growth. Members of this elite group secured great influence among European intellectual elites, American industrialists and colonial entrepreneurs. Development across the lifespan in this particular chronosystem would certainly present a unique worldview filled with opportunities for free non-conforming thinkers to thrive through unrestricted inquiry (Musson & Robinson, 1969; Strager, 2014).

Born in England in 1809, Charles Darwin provided the world with some of the original theories of evolution and natural selection. They would lay the foundation for most modern theories of evolutionary scientific inquiry. Darwin was well schooled, well-traveled and from a legacy of scholars, physicians, businessmen, artisans and abolitionists. His paternal grandfather Erasmus Darwin and maternal grandfather Josiah Wedgewood were both leading members of the Lunar Society and noted slave trade abolitionists. Charles Darwin would publish *On the Origin of Species* in 1859 which details his observations on the manner through which populations of organisms and their genes evolve over time through a process of natural selection. As he explains it, natural selection occurs when different genetic and phenotypic traits of organisms are favored by the ecosystems in which they develop. Those traits that are favored are sustained while those that are not fail to be passed on to future generations of organisms in that community. Charles Darwin benefitted from the work of his predecessor's, including his grandfathers. Thought leaders in the Lunar Society paved the road for his theories to be both developed and entertained where those in previous generations expressing non-religious-driven origin narratives were vilified, ex-communicated and/or hanged. Darwin's research would fuel many different factions of thought and robust research studies to develop new theories and innovative practices. The ideologies and paradigms born of extensions from this work were diverse; some were pro-social opportunities for growth and development while others would work to disenfranchise, disable and destroy (Bergman, 2014; Musson & Robinson, 1969; Strager, 2014).

Eugenics is derived from the Greek word eu—meaning good or well—and the suffix—genos meaning family or offspring—translating to well born or more colloquially and operationally to mean of good stock or noble race. Eugenics is grounded in efforts aimed at improving the quality of the human genetic community by eliminating and/or severely limiting the ability of 'non-desirable humans' to reproduce and populate future generations with their genes. Those who support eugenics—then and now—believe that conditions and characteristics like mental illness, race, criminality, poverty and "feeblemindedness" were genetically linked and passed down through biological means from parent to progeny. Although the construct of selective mating in human populations was not new, the term eugenics wasn't born until 1883 with the publication of *Inquiries into Human Faculty and Its Development* by British scientist Francis Galton (Bergman, 2014; Turda & Weindling, 2007).

Sir Francis Galton was born in 1822 and is responsible for advances across a wide variety of content areas. Through his contributions and 300-plus publications in statistics and math, biology, psychology and meteorology, he was a formidable surveyor and creator of knowledge. It is likely that Galton reflected upon his family lineage and determined that he was in fact from "good stock". He was considered a child prodigy, his grandfathers were abolitionists and his father was a scientist. Both Galton's paternal grandfather—Samuel Galton, a Quaker gun-manufacturer—and maternal grandfather, Josiah Wedgewood—also Charles Darwin's grandfather—were members of the Lunar Society. His cousin, Charles Darwin, was highly influential in the development of his theory of eugenics (Murdoch, 2007; Musson & Robinson, 1969; Strager, 2014). Most people are familiar with the concept of eugenics as it relates to the Nazi party and the efforts of Adolf Hitler to rid the world of people whom he had determined non-desirable, particularly those of Jewish descent. Hitler's eugenic framework manifested itself barbarically against Jewish and Romani families, incurably ill people, gay men and prisoners of war in the Holocaust. As a result, millions of people would die across the first half of the 1940s.

In 1933, Hilarius Gilges was abducted by Nazi officers in his hometown of Düsseldorf, Germany. Gilges was one of many mixed race Afro-Germans pejoratively referred to as "The Rhineland Bastards" by the Nazis. Hitler believed that Jewish people systematically brought Africans into the Rhineland to "pollute" their White Aryan blood line (Lusane, 2002; Oduah, 2016). French African colonial troops along with other

French and British soldiers occupied the German Rhineland which was to be left as a demilitarized zone after their departure. Once the war was over, as is often the case in war zones, there were children born of relationships that occurred during the occupation. The children of the Afro-French colonial soldiers represent some of the first generations of Afro-Germans to remain in the country, grow to numerable communities and raise their children alongside their fellow countrymen (Lusane, 2002).

Gilges was a performance artist, anti-Nazi labor organizer and communist. Black participation in the fight against Nazism and fascism in Eastern Europe is often ignored or overlooked. Although their numbers were small, there were non-immigrant Afro-Germans targeted for elimination and sterilization by Hitler and his party. When the Nazi party took power in the Rhineland region, Gilges—husband and father of two—was taken from his home, brutally tortured and subsequently murdered. His "brutalized and battered" body was found under the Rhineland bridge the same day of his abduction (Lusane, 2002).

Many are unfamiliar with the history of scientific racism against Black people across the diaspora that was often operationalized in Social Darwinism and eugenics across generations during and long after the start of the Transatlantic Slave Trade. When the macrosystemic features of the world have situated themselves to directly and indirectly, deliberately and inadvertently vilify an entire ethno-gender group, it must diversify the efforts that contribute to its demise. The efforts employed as a result of the discipline of eugenics are, although not likely intentional, several of many ways social and biological Darwinism live in the world (Bergman, 2014; Davidson, 1997). Energies from multi-disciplinary global factions contribute to these efforts through a system of structural racism that aims to consistently reduce opportunities for the genes of this specific group to be passed into future generations. Analyzed semantically, it appears clear that the murders of Black men by law enforcement, malevolent intergenerational academic practices, pathways that disproportionately lead to institutionalization, the promotion of environments that engender violence and poverty, government experimentation resulting in sterilization and the deliberate over exposure to toxins and substances of abuse all contribute to the general goals of eugenics: the reduction of the potentiality of a group's survival into future generations in general and their ability to mix with the group identified as dominant.

In 1904, Frederick Hertz—an Austrian-born, British naturalized sociologist and scholar—wrote *Modrne Rassentheorien* (Modern Race

Theories) and Antisemitismus und Wissenchaft (Anti-Semitism and Science). These works were published at the turn of the century, just as the construct of eugenics was growing in popularity. As the construct began gaining a following, Hertz was illustrating that existing race theories were often disguised efforts purposed to dominate, oppress and exploit. Hertz would demonstrate both through publication and lecture that empirical evidence failed to support any genetically superior or inferior race. In 1925, against the backdrop of a more matured Eugenics Movement, he published *Rasse und Kultur*, later published in English as *Race and Civilization*. Hertz agreed that there were in fact physical differences between various races, but that those differences were not inextricably tied to psychology or human behavior. Hertz was able to align himself with a contingent of intellectuals fighting against the race-based theories used by the Nazi party to justify the persecution they perpetuated against Jewish families, before, during and after what has become known as the Jewish Holocaust. Nazis and other oppressive groups used Darwinism alongside pseudo-theories to justify the performing of involuntary abortions and sterilizations on countless individuals for whom procreation was considered undesirable (Davidson, 1997; Lusane, 2002; Turda & Weindling, 2007). Today, very few people would feel comfortable discussing eugenics publically. Contemporary factors, however, create similar eugenic outcomes aimed at restricting the successful proliferation of populations deemed unfavorable. Some might argue that the murders of unarmed Black men by security and police, the strategic school to prison pipelines, the involuntary sterilizations and government initiated and/or sanctioned exposure to communicable diseases, toxins and substances of abuse are all ways in which eugenics is operationalized today.

It is neither secret nor coincidence that American police shoot and kill more people than their counterparts in other developed nations. A study in the Journal of American Medicine found that the US rate of gun deaths was 10.6 per 100,000 people in 2016 compared to the UK with a rate of 0.3 per 100,000 (Hamlin, 2018; Lopez, 2018). One causal factor in this extremely disparate rate is the average number of privately owned guns in each country. Simply put, more guns per person statistically creates more opportunities for gun violence. This is an inarguable mathematical fact. According to the 2017 Small Arms Study, there were one billion firearms in circulation around the globe. Of those weapons, 85% are owned by civilians and 2% by law enforcement (Small Arms Survey, 2018). In the USA, it is estimated that there were 120.5 guns for every 100 residents of the country in 2017. Yemen came in second with 52.8 guns, Canada fifth with 34.7 and France in twenty-second with 19.6 guns per 100 residents (Hamlin, 2018; Lopez, 2018).

The disproportionate rate with which Black men are murdered by law enforcement officers in the USA when compared to other countries is reflective of the equally as large disparity in overall gun violence and number of guns owned by civilians in each country. The fact that fewer Black men in the UK, France and Canada are murdered by police officers often leads people to believe that these men are not experiencing regular racist assaults at varying degrees of intensity just like US Black men. The truth is, Black men in each of these countries report strikingly similar experiences across the continuum of racist and racial encounters.

The Independent Office for Police Conduct reported that 47% of the people who died either in or following British police custody where force was used in 2017–2018 were Black (Independent Office of Police Conduct, 2018). This type of disproportionality is often minimized as a result of the shooting deaths in America. The true statistics of these American deaths is actually reflective of disparate gun availability in these nations and not disparate experiences with individual, interpersonal and institutional racism aimed at Black men. Our current perspective creates a false fissure between these men whose global healing might be catalyzed with a more cohesive understanding of a common lived experience among those in the diaspora living on lands dominated by White Eurocentric cultural norms.

In 2015, Andrew Loku, a 45-year-old Black Canadian father of five with a history of mental illness, was murdered by Toronto police officer Constable Andrew Doyle. One hour before he was shot in his apartment complex, Loku had been stopped by other officers while riding his electric bicycle on the highway. Court records indicate that officers transported Loku to his apartment after confiscating his bicycle because he appeared confused and under the influence of alcohol. Shortly after being dropped off at his apartment, a neighbor called authorities indicating that Loku was threatening residents and wielding a hammer. Audio of the July 2015 incident demonstrates that Loku, for over four minutes with hammer in hand, yelled and made alleged threats throughout the hallway without injury to self or others (DiManno, 2017; The Canadian Press, 2017).

In his closing arguments, Loku's family's attorney Jonathan Shime stated: "They shot him because they let their fear of a Black man with a hammer (8.5 meters away) overcome what should have been a compassionate and humane response." When officers arrived on the scene, Doyle was first up the stairs, followed by his "coach officer". Doyle commanded Loku to drop the hammer at a minimum of two times. After almost five minutes of neighbors experiencing the hammer wielding man, he remained alive. Only 19 seconds after Doyle's final command to drop the hammer, Loku lay dead from a bullet wound in his apartment complex hallway. In Canada, the police murders of Black men like Andrew Loku, Jermaine Carby and others continue to create chilling disparities in Canadian communities (DiManno, 2017; Gillis, 2015; The Canadian Press, 2017).

The twentieth century would end with the 1999 murder of Amadou Diallo in New York by four plain-clothes officers. Nineteen of the 41 bullets discharged from their firearms would impel themselves into him. Diallo was 23, had lived all around the world and was mistaken for a New York serial rapist (Fasick & Steinbuch, 2015). In 2005, Abou Bakari Tandia died in Courbevoie near Paris while in police custody following an identity check. As he lay comatose in a hospital room guarded by police officers, his family was denied the right to see him until the next day after receiving several conflicting stories as to the cause of his death (Le Parisien, 2011). Mark Duggan, a 29-year-old father, was murdered by British police in Tottenham, north London in 2011 for suspicion of illegal firearm possession (BBC, 2015; The Guardian, 2015). In 2012, 17-year-old high school junior Trayvon Martin was murdered by a community watchman in Florida for not complying with his orders as he walked to his father's fiancés home (CNN, 2018). Thirty-three-year-old Jermaine Carby, a passenger in a vehicle pulled over for drunk driving concerns, was killed in 2014 by an officer in Brampton, Ontario. Self-defense was used as justification for killing Carby due to an alleged knife he threatened officers with. No knife was ever found at the actual scene by investigators, but there was one presented by officers at a later time (City News, 2016). In Dalston, East London, 20-year-old Rashan Charles died after swallowing a package during a police foot chase which ended in 2017 with him being subdued by an officer who admittedly ignored several training protocols while a nearby citizen assisted in the restraint and detainment (Taylor, 2018). Twenty-two-year-old Aboubakar Fofana was killed by French police in Nantes, France, in 2018 after being under surveillance as a part of a drug trafficking investigation. The officer initially indicated that the shooting was in self-defense and later changed his story calling the shooting an accident (Willsher, 2018).

Although records from the first two decades of the twenty-first century document strong evidence of disproportionately excessive and fatal force aimed at Black men from the law enforcement community, it is critical to note that law enforcement agents across the globe are engaged in a career path that presents invariable and unpredictable dangers at every juncture. Supporting the safety of the world's communities and the people that make them great is neither easy nor safe, and the professionals trained to do so shoulder a massive set of responsibilities.

Law enforcement agents like all other professionals across the globe are impacted by the toxins of the world, including those that create a narrative of danger surrounding both the general existence and specific presence of Black men and boys. The duties associated with one's professional role will dictate the facet of structural racism in which biases manifest themselves. For instance, if you are a hotel manager, your victim might look like Jermaine Massey who was kicked out of a Portland hotel in December of 2018. He was making a phone call (to his mom) in the lobby of the hotel when approached by a security officer and told that he presented a threat to the other guests in the hotel. Even after showing his room keycard, the police were called and he was escorted off the property. Double Tree posted on social media that they fired the employees involved and were working with diversity experts "to ensure this never happens again" (Allen, 2018).

If you are a high school wrestling referee, your victim might look like New Jersey's 16-year-old Andrew Johnson. Forced to cut his dreadlocks off moments before a December 2018 wrestling match after being given 90 seconds to decide whether to cut his hair or forfeit the match. The referee, Alan Maloney—who had been recently accused of calling a Black colleague a "nigger" during a small gathering of wrestling officials—oversaw the trainer tasked to cut Johnson's hair. Maloney gave approval to participate in the match only after he determined that the length of Johnson's hair met league requirements. The New Jersey Wrestling Officials Association determined that the incident didn't rise to the level of terminating Maloney, who is reported to have volunteered to attend alcohol awareness and sensitivity training programs as his reprimand (Hohman, 2018). There are countless ways in which we see the treatment of Black men and boys informed and driven by generations of evolving narratives that support the myth of an inherent and intrinsic "danger nucleotide" sequenced into their DNA.

In 2011, Amnesty International published "France: Our lives are left hanging families of victims of deaths in police custody wait for justice to be done." The authors indicate: "Although persons of different ages, social backgrounds and nationalities are victims of human rights violations by law enforcement officials, the overwhelming majority of the cases brought to Amnesty International's attention concern persons belonging to ethnic minorities (Amnesty International, 2011, p. 5). The families of the five victims interviewed for the briefing had two major themes in common. They and their slain loved one were all ethnic minorities and they all described how the death of their loved one was made overwhelmingly worse due to a lack of justice, a shield of untruths and/or a lack of reparations, defined in the document as efforts aimed to "as far as possible, wipe out all the consequences of the illegal act and re-establish the situation which would, in all probability, have existed if the act had not been committed" (Amnesty International, 2011, p. 6). The underlying goal of this document is to tell a story, a first person narrative from the relatives of persons who died in police custody. It illustrates their common experiences that include an inadequate dedication of investigatory resources into the death of their family member, a lack of urgency given to the investigations that occur and a more realistic picture into the actual nature and scope of the obstacles faced in their efforts to seek truth and justice.

On his 24th birthday, Adama Traoré was riding his bike through Beaumont-sur-Oise, just north of Paris, to meet his older brother. When he and his brother were approached by police seeking his brother in connection to another case, he fled. Two hours later, he was found dead in the courtyard of a French police station. French officials provided an array of reasons for his death. Initial reports indicated that he died of heart disease, followed by reports of a serious infection attacking his internal organs. It was also reported that he had been drinking and smoking marijuana before his arrest. After a lengthy battle to access the body, Traoré's family was able to have an independent expert assess the cause of death. This review found no signs of heart disease, no infection and no signs of intoxicants. It was concluded that Traoré died of asphyxiation. Officers later admitted that he complained of having trouble breathing while denying that they had used any excessive force (Diallo, 2017; Graber, 2017).

The unreasonable deadly force used against Black men across the globe is alarming but not surprising as it remains fixed within a running schema that dictates how Black men and boys must be engaged across all arenas, including that of justice for crimes and the enforcement of laws. Independent of the training and philosophies that underpin how the law is enforced in a given municipality, the role of an officer is to maintain public safety and order while preventing, investigating and detecting criminal activity. As a result, this call of duty is wrought with opportunities for biases to operationalize themselves in the most fatal and traumatic of ways. A history of eugenics and social Darwinism has contributed to the strength of explicit and implicit biases that make the actual lives of Black men and boys more dispensable than others. Between 1882 and 1968, there were 3347 documented lynchings of Americans who were most all Black people (NAACP, 2016). Like other paradigms of oppression, modern-day murders of Black men for non-compliance demonstrate a newly fashioned noose, with comparable outcomes for each new generation it finds itself in. To state this point more deliberately, White people who engage in similar forms of non-compliance—and they do—are less likely to die at the hands of or in the custody of the agent.

Due to discourse on the expendability of the Black body and the life that inhabits it, unprincipled researchers and immoral organizations (public, private and government) have subjected Blacks to some very horrific experiences in the name of science and entertainment. Demeaning circus displays, debilitating syphilis experiments, unethical dissections and autopsies, experimental exposure to radiation, investigational live lobotomies and unauthorized sterilizations have all been used to assault Black bodies, both living and dead. In 2006, Harriet A. Washington published *Medical Apartheid: The Dark History of Medical Experimentation on Black Americans from Colonial Times to the Present*. In this text, the author explores a history of violations on Black bodies by the scientific and medical communities of unwilling, non-consenting and uninformed participants (Washington, 2006).

Given contemporary policies and laws regarding the protection of human subjects, it is hard for some to believe that individuals might have been treated so brutally. The construct of informed consent was non-existent during this time. It would not be introduced into the American lexicon until the late 1950s. Enslaved people were loaned to doctors for experimentation or even sold directly for the purposes of "research". Many medical procedures were practiced and perfected on Black people prior to being used on Whites for similar ailments.

American Slavery As It Is: Testimony of a Thousand Witnesses (1839) by Theodore Dwight Weld provided an early look into the dangers that medical science brought to the enslaved men and women. Weld was a significant figure in the abolitionist movement as we know it today. In the 1839 book, first-hand accounts of events are told from an array of voices represented in the varied communities. One account reflects on a college catalog describing the advantages of the South Carolina Medical College of Charleston.

A major factor of success as a medical doctor across specialties is a keen understanding and mastery of anatomy and physiology. South Carolina Medical College of Charleston boasted their "great opportunities for the acquisition of anatomical knowledge". By most accounts, a medical school that had these enriching anatomy and physiology core strengths would promote them to increase student enrollment and ensure adequate preparation for the medical field. In order to ensure there was no ambiguity, the document further read, "subjects being obtained from among the colored population in sufficient number for every purpose, and proper dissection carried out without offending any individuals in the community" (Weld, 1839, p. 169). Black corpses would be sold—without consent—to medical schools and science laboratories across the world to be butchered in the name of science and experimentation. It was common practice across the USA for people to raid Black cemeteries, steal corpses and sell them to medical and other more nefarious groups. The underpinning theory surrounding donating one's body for medical and scientific research is not the concern in this instance, it is both noble and valuable when approval is provided. The illegal pirating of Black bodies without the consent of the individual or the family speaks to a dismissal of humanity that would be used to justify not only the abuse of the Black corpse but the Black body that still held life with hopes, dreams and emotions. It is estimated that upward of 5000 cadavers were dissected each year during this time period in the USA and that most of them were acquired through illegal means (Clark, 1998).

In 1980, the World Health Assembly affirmed that the world had been freed from small pox, a deadly disease that ravished communities across centuries. In 1796, British doctor Edward Jenner discovered that by introducing a similar virus from cows into people, the risk for contracting small pox fell drastically. Jenner worked with Harvard professor Benjamin Waterhouse (Washington, 2006; Williams, 2010) in attempts to mainstream the process in the USA. Waterhouse would reach out to planter and scientist Thomas Jefferson who had long been performing dangerous inoculations on non-consenting enslaved Blacks at Monticello and neighboring plantations. Although there is conjecture regarding the actual individuals used in his nineteenth-century clinical trials, evidence seems to demonstrate that he exposed hundreds of enslaved men and women to these dangerous viruses in order to assess its safety before disseminating to White peers (Washington, 2006; Williams, 2010).

After bacteriologists in France began to advance the research on infectious diseases, the populations to experiment on were sought after. Prisoners and children who had been left abandoned were often the subjects of trials in France and England. Typhoid fever was a disease with a history of ravishing communities across the globe. Dr. Walter E. Jones of Petersburg, Virginia, documented an experiment where he would pour boiling water onto the naked back of a 25-year-old enslaved man at four-hour intervals to treat symptoms of the disease. His hypothesis had no significant evidence behind its query, but the lack of value placed upon the man's life skewed the cost–benefit ratio (Washington, 2006).

The manipulated cost to benefit analysis would be further skewed with James Marion Sims, often celebrated as the father of modern gynecology. Born in 1813 in South Carolina, he eventually became a southern plantation doctor and surgeon servicing enslaved Blacks and the families of their enslavers in Montgomery, Alabama. In one case, while working at the South Carolina Medical College, Dr. Sims performed surgery on an unsuspecting enslaved man forced into the procedure by his owner after becoming unproductive on the plantation. The enslaved man named Sam, after being invited to sit with Sims, was ambushed by young doctors who bound him with straps at almost every joint from his ankles and feet to his head and shoulders. Once the man was immobilized, over 20 people, including medical students and curious on-lookers, filed in to watch as Sims removed a large portion of the unwilling patient's lower jawbone without anesthesia (Brown, 2017; Wall, 2006; Washington, 2006).

Sims' observations of high infant mortality rates among enslaved women led to a host of presumptions including poverty, blunted moral and social feelings, and laziness that blamed the women for the deaths of their infants. By the mid-1800s, he was a beloved and popular local figure with a thriving practice. Between 1845 and 1849, Sims would conduct extensive, invasive experimental surgeries on 12 enslaved women in a small hospital he built for these studies. These women, often suffering from pre-existing gynecological concerns, were placed under Sims' care at his request. It is alleged that when one owner refused the terms of the experimentation, Sims simply purchased her (Wall, 2006; Washington, 2006).

The widely held belief during this time that Black people didn't experience pain fueled these experiments of unanaesthetized trauma when the inhalation of ether as an anesthetic had been in use, although not widely, since the 1840s. It is reported that the enslaved women were forced to hold one another down during these torturous events after Sims' peers abandoned the project due to an inability to tolerate the shrieks of agony accompanying each procedure. These types of events were neither unusual nor relegated to one doctor in South Carolina.

Sims would later learn, along with the remainder of the medical community, that the presumptions which informed much of his work on these patients were wrong. Enslaved women and the children he experimented on did in fact feel pain. Infants of the enslaved were dying because of the slave quarters proximity to livestock, its waste and the microbial profile associated. Finally, many of the other diseases observed in infants and toddlers would be the result of malnutrition and vitamin deficiencies common to the diet of enslavement. After Sims mastered his surgeries by mutilating the vaginas of Black women, he moved to New York and opened a women's hospital where he performed the surgery on White women with anesthetic and a set of skills that rendered him expertly competent by this time (Brown, 2017; Washington, 2006).

In the late nineteenth century, syphilis had been identified as a major health threat among southern Blacks. Racist paradigms and motivations of medical professionals in the absence of scientific evidence would prevail to use racial stereotypes like "excessive sexual desire, immorality, large penises and small brains" to explain disease prevalence. This philosophy would open the door to the American calamity known as the Tuskegee Syphilis Study initiated in 1932 by the United States Public Health Service (USPHS) in Macon County, Alabama. The goal of the government study was to track the course of untreated syphilis in Black men. Three hundred ninety-nine men with syphilis and 201 uninfected men made up the sample of participants recruited from local churches and clinics with the promise of free meals, special treatment for "bad blood" and burial insurance (Bernal, 2013; The Tuskegee Experiment, 2015).

Nurse Eunice Rivers, a graduate of Tuskegee Institute, and Dr. Eugene H Dribble, medical director of John A. Andrew Memorial Hospital, were the practitioners identified by the USPHS to run the study. Rivers was born in 1899 in rural Georgia and graduated from Tuskegee Institute's School of Nursing in 1922, just as precursors to the Great Depression began to dismantle the economic structure of the nation. Booker T. Washington created the Movable School—his public health initiative—to improve the living conditions and education of poor rural farmers.

Rivers became a trusted figure throughout the Black farming communities of Tuskegee and the surrounding areas due to her traveling work with the college's adult education-focused Movable School, providing curricula that included agriculture, health and home economics. She taught families how to make bandages from old clothing, improve sanitation to prevent disease, care for sick loved ones and even prevent sexually transmitted infections. She would later move from work with the Alabama Bureau of Child Welfare to the Bureau of Vital Statistics where she worked to reduce infant mortality through improved regulations and training for southern midwives. She even trained children on dental hygiene, providing them with tubes of toothpaste provided by the company (Bernal, 2013; The Tuskegee Experiment, 2015).

Her role within this Black rural community included some of the most intimate of professional to consumer spaces in existence. Trust has the capacity to grow exponentially in these spaces. After building such a high level of social capital throughout her career, it was not coincidental that she would be identified and selected to be consumer facing ambassador of destruction. There exists an array of opinions that both vilify and support Rivers by contextualizing her actions in the space and time they occurred. It is unclear how much she knew about the actual nature of the study. Some say that because she is listed as the author on several of the papers that she certainly knew what was happening. Others state that she was simply a pawn of American medical racism operationalized in the south. It may never be possible to know the answers to what she knew and didn't, but we can be clear on several significant outcomes of this experiment (Bernal, 2013; The Tuskegee Experiment, 2015).

The USPHS knew that Rivers had built trust throughout this community and that she would be effective at maximizing study participation. The participants she recruited who already had syphilis were denied treatment, even after penicillin had been approved for treatment in 1947. The study lasted a full 40 years resulting in generations of families negatively impacted by their father's, husband's, grandfather's or great-grandfather's experience as one of the 600 men studied without knowing the full extent of the study. Researchers and study facilitators, including Rivers, insisted that participants remain in the study even when they had learned that a cure was found that didn't include the toxicity and danger of the previous remedies like Salvarsan and Neosalvarsan (Bernal, 2013; The Tuskegee Experiment, 2015).

In 1972, the Associated Press broke the story of the Tuskegee Experiment resulting in cessation of the study and the initiation of an Ad Hoc Advisory Panel. Public outcry was heavy over the 40-year experiment that had been cloaked to the public but spoken openly about in medical circles across the country. As late as 1969, a committee at the US Centers for Disease Control (CDC) investigated the study and authorized its continuance. In 1997, US President Bill Clinton invited the remaining experiment survivors to the White House for a public apology. Herman Shaw, Charlie Pollard, Carter Howard, Frederick Moss and Fred Simmons all well into their 90s and beyond listened as President Clinton apologized. "The American people are sorry for the loss, for the years of hurt. You did nothing wrong, but you were grievously wronged. I apologize and I am sorry that this apology has been so long in coming." The families of the survivor's report that they continue to experience the intergenerational traumas associated with the details of the assault on their families (Ross, 2017).

The use of the Black body for medical experimentation is thought to have catalyzed the cannon of American medical knowledge once the practices began crossing the Atlantic from Europe. Enslaved people had no choice, and post-emancipation Blacks were often led into medical experimentation by deception and trickery. All across the country, Black bodies were displayed and paraded for science and entertainment, dissected for random exploration and experimentation or operated on to test non-scientific hypotheses. Much of this history remains hidden or re-envisioned by white-washed narratives that mystify the exponential growth of knowledge exposure and wealth at the expense of Black bodies (Washington, 2006).

In 2017, The Greatest Showman, a musical about the life and success of famed circus entrepreneur P.T. Barnum, was released worldwide. Barnum born in 1810 was a small business owner and a Connecticut legislator before becoming an American showman. Critics of the film were concerned with some of the film's historical gaps that failed to mention his production of southern minstrel shows or how his rise to fame was on the back of an elderly enslaved woman who he leased for $1000 a year. Joice Heth was a blind and largely paralyzed woman who was inaccurately billed as the 161-year-old wet nurse of George Washington. Heth would be exhibited in Barnum's touring displays for 10–12 hours each day until she died in 1836, when he would truly make his mark as a showman.

As Barnum worked throughout the American northeast, he assured his followers and fans that once Heth died, he would have a public autopsy of her body to prove her age. He of course knew that she was not 161 years old but was sure that people would pay to see the body of a Black woman dissected and mutilated for entertainment purposes. He was right: he charged 50 cents per person for the people of New York to have a front row seat at the table of ultimate dispensability, a public dismantling for entertainment with no provision of scientific or humanistic benefits to society. Like so many others, Heth was another representation of how race science and eugenics have laid the groundwork for a visceral intergenerational perspective on the nature and value of the Black body (Mansky, 2017; Washington, 2006).

School Nooses

Education and academic programs in most industrialized nations tend to be structured around a model that we typically attribute to ancient Greek philosophers like Thales, Socrates, Aristotle and Pythagoras. The foundations of math, language arts, history and communication have been attributed to these men often without question. Greek men, categorically credited with developing the foundations of modern academia, once sat at the feet of African priests and priestesses. The record of Kemetic history demonstrates millennia of library science that included astronomy and astrology, geography and geology, philosophy, theology, law and communication.

In the tombs of Neb-Nufre and Nufre-Hetep—father and son library priests—bearing the titles of *her schâtu* (Superior over the Books) and *naa en schâtu* (Chief over the Books) were royal sacrifices and evidence of pre-existing libraries and a system of academia that supported its development. Herodotus, in reference to the Egyptians, stated that they were "by far the best instructed people with whom he has become acquainted, since they, of all men, store up most, for recollection" (Lepsius, 1853, p. 383). Danus, Archimedes, Herodotus and Plato all studied in Egypt prior to returning to Europe with the knowledge they gained while studying, some for decades, with the Africans. People often deny one of two facts related to these evidences. They either "other" the Egyptians and Ethiopians by making them "not African" or they erroneously deny the Grecian travels to Africa. Aristotle, in Physiognomonica—an exposition on the practice of assessing one's character from outward appearance—wrote "the Ethiopians and Egyptians are very Black". Herodotus adds that the Egyptians had "Black skin and wooly hair". Prototypes of "mathematics, medicine, astronomy, metallurgy, philosophy, religion and the arts" (Finch, 1987) that predate Greek attribution were unearthed when scientists and loot-ers began to excavate ancient burial grounds. Cheikh Anta Diop and other noted Egyptologists challenged the white washing of the Egyptians and worked to ensure people knew they were in fact Black Africans and not White Europeans. Although literal documentation of libraries and learned communities in Thebes, Luxor, Alexandria, Abydos and beyond exist across African antiquity, the thematic perception of academia's grounding in Eurocentric Grecian tradition continues to prevail (James, 1954; Lepsius, 1853). These narratives generate a dangerous paradigm as Black children experience stereotype threat and disidentification in response to an ecology that tells them that academic prowess is not their birthright.

In a 2015 French survey, the Organization for Economic Co-operation and Development found that French student's social, economic and cultural backgrounds had the greatest impact on school performance when compared to the other 70 countries in the study. In the study, only 2% of the country's top performers were from low-income backgrounds which like most other Euronormative nations are often highly racialized. A disproportionate reliance upon geographic and socio-economic data to inform policy on social inequity, like in France, is known to negatively impact valuable utility of data collected. Although France is not completely ignoring ecological factors that cre-ate indirect racial and ethnic disparity, they seem to remain reluctant to the idea of collecting race-specific data. The French Educational Priority Zones (ZEP) initiative, where additional resources are allocated to under-resourced schools that tend to matriculate immigrant and minor-ity students has seen some success, but fails to address the broader con-cern that remains when one controls for socio-economic status. (Chhor, 2016).

In 2018, The Challenge, a non-profit organization in the UK, found that data from over 20,000 schools revealed varying degrees of race/ethnic and socio-economic segregation across the country. In many cases the race segregation within schools continued to exist even when students lived in neighborhoods that were not highly segregated. Jon Yates, the organiza-tion's director at the time of the study, stated that, "when communities live separately, anxiety and prejudice flourish, whereas when people from differ-ent backgrounds mix, it leads to more trusting and cohesive communities and opens up opportunities for social mobility" (The Challenge, 2017).

Evidence demonstrates that the segregation of children contributes to mistrust and ultimately to intolerance of others. The report cited decades of research showing the scope of segregation in schools in the UK (The Challenge, 2017, The Challenge; Coughlan, 2015).

In the USA, not only were Black children not welcome in schools, anti-literacy laws made it a punishable crime to educate them. Once afforded access to formal education, the question of segregation saturated the American and Canadian academic settings where the practice was legal. Ontario was a Canadian nucleus for Blacks escaping enslavement. Although laws failed to segregate Canadian school systems, segregated schools existed in cities like Windsor and Chapman in addition to cities in other provinces across the country. The last segregated school in Canada—Nova Scotia—was closed in 1983 (Historic Canada).

From the past of anti-literacy legislation, to multi-generational academic disenfranchisement, to the contemporary school to institutionalization pathways, schools have consistently served as the backdrop for structural injuries of a racist nature against Black children. These injuries are often correlated with a component of oversight by an institution or government organization. From living in a congregate care home for juveniles labeled as emotionally disturbed to sitting on death row awaiting the verdict of your final appeal, the foundation set by early education plays a formidable role in one's trajectory. In addition to segregated and under-resourced schools, a critical component of these aforementioned injuries has been the developmental damage done by the over utilization of intelligence assessments on Black children as a tool to determine the factors of academic settings that make them either least restrictive or most inclusive.

Cognitive performance, acuity and aptitude have historically been assessed using intelligence tests. Intelligence Quotient (IQ) was coined by German psychologist William Stern and determined by comparing an individual's "mental age" as demonstrated on a standardized test, to their chronological age. The construct of IQ would later be used by other researchers to develop and refine the intelligence tests they would come to develop. One of the most widely used intelligence test, the Stanford–Binet Intelligence Scales, was developed in France by psychologist Alfred Binet and revised by Stanford University psychologist Lewis Terman for use on American populations. The most current edition of the test uses five scales—knowledge, quantitative reasoning, visual spatial processing, working memory and fluid reasoning—to diagnose intellectual deficiencies and developmental deficits in school-aged children (Leslie, 2000; Murdoch, 2007).

As the administration of intelligence tests for children widened, Terman became a staunch advocate for the use of standardized testing to categorize individuals and tailor educational supports, services and career tracks to their scores. The US government soon took notice and asked that he create another assessment tool to be used by the US military. This assessment tool would assign a quantifiable intelligence measurement to soldiers in order to determine whether a man would enter their branch of service as an officer or not. Terman became the face and voice of the standardized testing machine that would spread with endemic speeds, largely unquestioned (Murdoch, 2007).

Black historian and theorist Horace Man Bond saw the concerns with intelligence testing and its misuse in education settings very clearly. In 1972, he wrote:

> … ever since the "measurement of minds" became a popular field in which to pursue investigations, the testing of Negro children has easily ranked as a major indoor sport among psychologists … The rules of the game are simple and seem to be standardized throughout the country with but few exceptions. First one must have a *White* examiner; a group of *Negro* children; a test standardized for *White* children tested by *White* examiners; and just a few pre-conceived notions regarding the nature of "intelligence" and the degree to which Negro children are endowed if at all … and the *fact* that social status of Negro children need not be considered as an extra allowance for scores different from Whites. (Winfield, 2007, p. 130)

In addition to his work on the development of the intelligence test, Terman was also responsible for initiating one of the longest longitudinal studies ever conducted. His research was published in 1925 as *Genetic Studies of Genius*. Considered groundbreaking at the time, it aggregated a group of traits, mechanisms and circumstances that dominant culture theorists used to explain what giftedness looked like. It later evolved to explain how intelligence influences measurable success outcomes in adulthood. In this study, Terman and his colleagues attempt to determine what traits differentiate the gifted child from the "typical child of normal mentality" by collecting data on over 1.400 youth within the top 1% of the of the school population. Terman's sample was overwhelmingly White, male and Californian; it included only two African Americans, six Japanese Americans and one Native American (Leslie, 2000; Murdoch, 2007).

Terman, like many of his contemporaries, was an intransigent hereditarian who openly endorsed practices of eugenics. The man who created the American version of the test that determined academic trajectory and military ranking was in fact one who also openly endorsed the need for people of lesser intelligence to be institutionalized and sterilized in order to ensure procreation by individuals with a higher aptitude for intelligence. Although critiques of this model were well articulated, by the 1930s IQ testing was prominent in the USA and children with higher IQs were being placed into more challenging classrooms in preparation for high paying jobs and college careers. Children who had lower scores on their tests received no academic enrichment and were bound by the self-fulfilling prophecy birthed of low expectations (Leslie, 2000; Murdoch, 2007; Winfield, 2007).

In his published study, Terman develops ecological conclusions that further illustrate his mission. In fact, his explanation tells a tale of how all children are actually provided equitable access to comparable education and enriching engagement from teachers and peers.

> Although a majority of our children (study participants) have had the advantage of superior cultural influences in the home, their more formal educational opportunities have been entirely commonplace, in no way superior to those enjoyed by the children from the humblest families in Los Angeles, San Francisco, and Oakland. At school, they have studied and played with the children of the generality. The school has provided for them no special program of instruction. It has given no form of individual treatment. (Terman, 1925, p. 636)

Terman became the face of standardized testing and the advocate for utilizing the results to create an American caste system cloaked in a meritocracy of false positives. Not only does Terman dismiss the differential treatment afforded to individuals based on their test results, he adds that—based on additional tests—gifted children also demonstrate higher degrees of moral traits like honesty and trustworthiness. By the mid-twentieth century, "ability tracks" based primarily upon the results of intelligence tests like the Stanford–Binet were utilized to situate children in classes with others of similar ability. Once placed into one of these tracks, it was virtually impossible for a child to be moved into another ability track.

Julius Hobson, born in Birmingham, AL, in 1922 worked in a library as a child; a library he was not allowed to borrow books from. He would go on to be a WWII army pilot, attend Tuskegee Institute, Columbia University and Howard University where he earned a graduate degree in economics. He strategically accessed leadership roles and membership in organizations like the National Association for the Advancement of Colored People (NAACP) and even became the president of the school's Parent Teachers Association. He gained national attention and was eventually hired by the Congress of Racial Equality (CORE), becoming an influential voice in desegregating restaurants, fighting employment discrimination and increasing housing equity. Hobson would be cast out of CORE in 1964 for becoming too radical for the pacifist lens that painted the organization's non-violent approach to addressing racial inequities (Wolters, 2008).

In 1965, Julius Hobson's 10-year-old daughter was placed into the lowest ability track at her school. Incensed and informed, he proceeded to sue the school district. Although Boiling v Sharpe (1954) ended legal school segregation in Washington, DC, the tracking systems relegated Black and poor children to academic tracks that denied them access to academic opportunities afforded to their White peers. This was common practice in many school systems around the world. In Hobson v Hansen (1967), he and other parents brought suit against the school district contending that the tracking system used was not based on ability and was moreover being used to promote segregation (Wolters, 2008).

Dr. Carl F. Hansen, the district's superintendent at the time, had based his entire educational philosophy on the system of ability tracking, including his own 1954 book, *The Four-track Curriculum in Today's High Schools*. Hobson's attorneys presented the court with data illustrating a strong correlation between: socio-economic status and academic performance tracks determined by aptitude tests, overcrowded Black schools and underpopulated White schools, racially restrictive teacher hiring and school assignment processes, and a disparate median annual per pupil expenditure between predominantly Black schools ($292 per student) and predominantly White school ($392 per students). The defendants acknowledged the data but denied that it was a manifestation of any racial bias or structural racism. In the end, the court ruled that the school district's policies denied equal opportunity to students, granting an injunction that led to the end of ability tracking in Washington DC schools

(Hallinan, 2000). Among the many principal findings in the opinion rendered by circuit court Judge J. Skelly Wright was this assault to aptitude testing:

> The aptitude tests used to assign children to the various tracks are standardized primarily on White middle class children. Since these tests do not relate to the Negro and disadvantaged child, track assignment based on such tests relegated Negro and disadvantage children to the lower tracks from which, because of the reduced curricula and the absence of adequate remedial and compensatory education, as well as continued inappropriate testing, the chance to escape is remote. (Justia US Law, 1967)

In 1970, Ray C. Rist wrote *Social Class and Teacher Expectations: Self-Fulfilling Prophecy in Ghetto Education* where he followed a group of kindergarten students to assess movement from the original ability groups they were placed into. He noted that the reading groups the children were placed in were reflective of the social class composition of the classroom and explored the specific risk factors impacting their growth and enrichment. One noteworthy observation from Rist's work was how children's achievement was influenced by the way the teacher behaved toward the different groups. This supports a host of literature pre-dating his publication that demonstrated, without fail, that the teacher's expectations of a child's performance had a strong influence on their actual performance. Shortly after this publication in 1974, the US Commission on Civil Rights found that 63% of elementary schools and 79% of secondary schools in five southwestern US states continued to use forms of ability grouping. They further found that "minorities were overrepresented in low ability-group classes, and underrepresented in high ability-group classes" (Brown, 2017, p. 479). In 1976, James Rosenbaum wrote *Making Inequality* where he described dangerous outcomes of the vocational and remedial tracks that working-class New England high school students were being placed into. "Tracking and ability grouping are not mere bystanders to social injustice … Such practices don't just mirror the inequalities of the broader society. They reproduce and perpetuate inequality" (Loveless, 2013, p. 15).

A report conducted by Carl James of York University found that huge disparities present inside schools in the Greater Toronto Area (GTA) continue to persist for Black students. The research found that Black students were being streamed into applied programs at a higher rate than

White students. According to the research, only 53% of Black student were being enrolled into academic programs when compared to 81% of their White counterparts (Canadian Broadcasting System [CBC], 2017). Almost 40% of all Black students in the sample were enrolled in applied programs when compared to 16% of White students, although "education streaming", a Canadian version of ability tracking, was outlawed in 1999 (Draaisma, 2017). The value and importance of applied programs of study and vocational curricula are well understood, and the goal here is to determine the etiology of the disparity and understand tools for its prevention, not to minimize the important spaces those programs fill.

Compounding this academic system of disenfranchisement and under-education is the fact that 42% of the Black student population had been suspended at least once. In addition, almost half of all the Toronto District School Board (TDSB) students suspended over a five-year period were also Black compared to the 10% who were White across this same time period (CBC, 2017; The Canadian Press, 2017). In response to the results of this study, TDSB executive superintendent Jim Spyropoulos acknowledged the systemic risk factors that impact students, stating: "Unless we start by addressing power and privilege and the bias that each one of us brings to our spaces each and every day, then I don't know we are ever going to be able to confront the problem" (The Canadian Press, 2017).

In *Larry P. v Riles* (1979), a group of California parents sued the school district for the use of intelligence testing that resulted in the disproportionate placement of Black children into classes for the "educable mentally retarded (EMR)". Opinions rendered in this case indicated that

> … the history of IQ testing and special education in California, reveals an unlawful segregative intent. This intent was not necessarily to hurt Black children, but it was an intent to assign a grossly disproportionate number of Black children to the special EMR classes, and it was manifested … in the use of unvalidated and racially and culturally biased placement criteria. This intent, consistent only with an impermissible and unsupportable assumption of a higher incidence of mental retardation among Blacks, cannot be allowed in the face of the constitutional prohibition of racial discrimination. (Larry P. v Riles, Supp 933)

These efforts have created a long-lasting framework that has disenfranchised and under-educated Black children for generations. In the 2008 National Assessment of Educational Progress, the reading scores of Black boys in eighth grade were only slightly higher than the scores of White girls in fourth grade. In this same study, 46% Black boys demonstrated math scores at a rating of "basic" or above compared to 82% of White boys (Kirp, 2010). In the 2018 Brown Center Report on American Education, the Brookings Institute reports that the US White–Black achievement gap in both math and reading as assessed by the National Assessment of Educational Progress (NAEP) has remained wide with little movement over the last decade (Hansen, Levesque, Valant, & Quintero, 2018). The Black–White achievement gap in the UK is certainly visible, although in *Coincidence or Conspiracy?*, English researcher David Gillborn contends that it is being effectively hidden by several major factors. A major contributor is the re-envisioning of White working-class boys as new race victims work to reconstruct the narrative of structural racism within the system of British education, while creating an imaginary educational system where only one group has the capacity to achieve at their highest potential. The UK has been disproportionately focusing on socio-economic status as an aggregate group to tell the story of their academic disparity (Gillborn, 2008).

Large-scale empirical studies report that "controls for socio-economic status typically reduce the Black-White gap by no more than one-third, and often by less, and that substantial gaps remain" (Strand, 2012, p. 4). Although poverty comes along with important academic risk factors to measure, it fails to accurately or adequately capture the differential experiences and needs of Black children across socio-economic strata, particularly when gaps persist. When all groups are disaggregated by race and gender, a more accurate set of outcomes show how structural components of academic systems do in fact impact Black children in very specific ways. Finally, selectively skewing actual data to misrepresent the real nature and scope of race inequality in the school systems promote a false perspective of actual needs and outcomes. In *Moving the Goal Post: Racial Segregation and the Black/White Achievement Gap, 1992–2009* (2017), British researchers found that over a 25-year period "White students were always at least one and a half times more likely to attain the dominant benchmark than their Black peers". They support a "sustained and explicit focus on race inequity in education policy" to best address the needs of all children (Gillborn, Demack, Rollock, & Warmington, 2017).

MECHANISTIC MEDIA

There is a plethora of media imagery that consistently illustrates Black men in unfavorable lights. Propaganda are selected messages and communications that often generalize characteristics of a group or condition to promote a particular agenda or viewpoint. Exploring the many images that bombard the world regarding Black men is critical. Research consistently demonstrates that "dehumanization is aroused, exacerbated, and exploited by propaganda" (Livingstone Smith, 2011) which can all work together to enhance an environment's capacity and propensity to injure. In a 2018 response to Canadian gun violence, Toronto Mayor John Tory called Afro-Canadian men "thugs and sewer rats" while city councilor Giorgio Mammoliti referred to them as criminals and cockroaches "who must be sprayed". This is unfortunately not unique as world leaders, government officials and public figures have consistently provided example after example of unrestricted vitriol against Black men (Kitossa, 2018).

The minstrel shows of American Reconstruction crystallized three major images of the newly and in some cases partially emancipated Black men: the Sambo, the Brute and the Zip Coon. Sambo was dedicated to singing and dancing to the contentment of White audiences. As a character in Uncle Tom's Cabin, he served as an overseer for Simon Legree and is ultimately responsible for killing Uncle Tom. The Brute appears consistently and was unfailingly in need of segregation and isolation to ensure the safety of communities and White citizens, White women in particular. Zip Coon was popularized by a song of the same name in the 1830s. Zip Coon was a Black face character that was a freedman who buffoonishly mimicked White upper-class speech and costume. These caricatures would be used to justify brutal systems of oppression on Black men. They signified the ways in which Black men have been degraded, demeaned and diminished. With all this evidence, even in the twenty-first century, people justify the use of Blackface in costumes for Halloween or for Eurocentric cultural celebrations.

St Nicholas Eve, December 5th, is a major nationwide celebration in Belgium and the Netherlands. It is a celebration of the next day's St Nicholas Day festivities. It is a day filled with the arrival of presents delivered by Sinterklaas (St Nicholas) and his team of Zwarte Piet. Zwarte Piet is a beloved character, central to celebrations of St. Nicholas Day. Also known as Black Pete, Zwarte Piet has been depicted in art and literature as a Black man with a curly/kinky hair texture common to many people of African descent, gold earrings and exaggerated lips. Historically, he has been described as ethnically Moorish, dressed in colorful garb with lace collars and ruffled sleeves. In Sinterklaas celebrations across Europe, hundreds of White Europeans move out into the parade streets in full Black face, paying deliberate homage to Black Pete and perhaps to a history of colonialism and enslavement on which their foundations of nationalism were built.

The Netherlands abolished slavery in 1863 after a long and detailed involvement. Based on survey results, the majority of the countries that celebrate this character don't see the image as representative of any racial stereotypes or general racism at all. Although most favor maintaining Black Pete just as he is, some have made some accommodations to his story, indicating that his skin is Black due to his travels up and down chimneys throughout the evening. Some have even moved to calling him Schoorsteen Piet or Chimney Pete. Children's Ombudsman in the Netherlands stated that the character of Zwarte Piet can contribute to bullying, exclusion or discrimination and is therefore in violation of the Convention on the Rights of the Child. In 2018, McDonald's Corporate office, after a social media post to its corporate social media page, banned employees from dressing up as Black Pete and the Dutch Police announced that Piet costumes would not be allowed in holiday parades after 2020 (Levelt, 2018). One Black man, an expat in Holland, described a Sinterklaas celebration as "perplexing and horrendous … much like being in the Twilight Zone" (Leeuwen, 2018).

Père Fouttard—the "Whipping Father" in France—is often depicted identically to Zwarte Piet. Each of these characters and many like them have origins in the delivery of punishment for "naughty children". In some tales, poorly behaved children were carried away to foreign lands in the bags of these dark men. In others they were spanked or given lumps of coal. As these contingents to rid Europe of Zwarte Piet grow, so do the White supremacist groups in favor of keeping him he as is. National Geographic News reports that journalists who have publically denounced Black Pete have received death threats and activists have been attacked by organized groups of White supremacists (Little, 2018). There is something substantive about such significant support for the maintenance of a practice that has been demonstrated to create harm and discomfort for a group of people.

Like the minstrel shows of the nineteenth century, twenty-first-century media across all modalities—television, film, print, web, video games, theater—continue to drive a narrative aimed to maintain Eurocentric dominance over Black men and boys. Both the over- and under- representation in media portrayals are striking. Black men are less likely than others to be a playable character in a video game (besides sports games), identified as a real life expert in news or documentaries or shown as a victim of violent non-race-based crimes. In addition, they are equally as rarely portrayed as involved in a parenting situation or engaged in intellectually positioned roles in works of fiction. For all the things that Black men are less likely to be across media, there are many more that they are more likely to be. Black men are over-represented as perpetrators of violent crimes, impoverished bystanders, members of fictitious criminal line-ups (or mugshot photos) and/or aggressors toward disproportionately White victims (The Opportunity Agenda).

Two of the most coveted awards for film actors across the globe are presented by the Academy of Motion Picture Arts and Sciences (Oscars) and the Screen Actors Guild (SAG). Both organizations operate out of Beverly Hills, CA, and usually host their annual award ceremonies in Los Angeles County. The awarded films, performances, artists and crew associated with them often represent what was, for that year, the gold standard. Actors are nominated for performances thought to be highly impactful or transformational. In many cases, the nominations and selected performances are a testament to the human reflex that resolves tensions and anxieties of dissonance without conscious effort. There is a reason why some performances from some actors are seen as groundbreaking and worthy of nomination. There is also a reason why one might feel exceedingly connected to how well the actor interpreted the script they were provided with.

The world has created an environment where Santa Claus, James Bond and Jesus, men who no one walking the Earth today has ever met, can *only* be White. The celebrated performances of Black men demonstrate a bifurcated effort to maintain centuries of strategic behaviors that maligned the images of Black men and provide them with consistent discursive injuries.

A rudimentary exploration of the aggregated Oscar and SAG awards data on the roles Black men (Wikipedia, Academy Awards; Wikipedia, Screen Actors Guild) have been celebrated for presents a stark reality that many have avoided over the years.

In the category of The Academy's Best Actor in a Leading Role, there have been 20 Black men nominated across 60 years between 1958 and 2018. Of these 20 nominations—representing 14 Black actors—a total of only four wins would be achieved for this high honor. Almost 40 years would pass between Sidney Poitier's win in 1963 and Denzel Washington's win in 2001. Less than a decade after the first honor was given, Poitier became the first Black actor to ever win the top award, Washington would be the second. In the category of Best Actor in a Supporting Role, there have been 17 nominations of Black men between 1969 and 2016 with a total of five wins across 15 actors. An aggregate total of nine wins across 37 nominations for Black actors nominated as either Best Actor or Best Supporting Actor across a 60-year period tells a story of disparity, while an examination of the content interpreted by the celebrated actor tells an even more important one.

The nine awarded actors were Sidney Poitier (1963), Loius Gossett Jr. (1982), Denzel Washington (1989 and 2001), Cuba Gooding Jr. (1996), Morgan Freeman (2004), Jamie Foxx (2004), Forest Whitaker (2006) and Mahershala Ali (2016). Each of these actor's performances rose to the level of excellence as their interpretation of the characters they were tasked to play—fictitious or real—translated to a monetized and emotional connection with audiences. An astute observer might wonder if these performances were so highly celebrated not only as a result of a stellar performance, but because the role selected for celebration fit a common archetype presented to the world about Black men.

In 1963, Sidney Poitier portrayed Homer Smith, the roaming handyman in *Lilies of the Field*. Smith becomes the singing Black savior for the Eastern European nuns attempting to build a chapel for their local congregation (a separate but equally as problematic archetype of European colonialism also saturates the nuns' approach to the local community). Smith is celebrated—although not compensated—for miraculously saving the community, teaching the nuns English and completing the construction of the chapel. In 1982, Louis Gossett Jr. was honored for his role as Emil Foley, a hard-nosed, no nonsense Marine sergeant in *An Officer and a Gentleman*. Foley is a homophobic, bellowing, paternalistic model of hyper-masculinity. In 1989, Denzel Washington won for his role as Private Trip, in *Glory*. Trip was a formerly enslaved man fighting in the American Civil War in an all-Black unit where he found family for the first time. He would go on to win in the best actor category in 2001 as Alonzo Harris, a power hungry, drug-addicted, dirty police officer in *Training Day*. In 1996, Rod Tidwell, Cuba Gooding Jr.'s football playing character, gave us the iconic "Show me the money!" catch phrase. In *Jerry Maguire*, Tidwell was a money-hungry, pretentious narcissist who was led to the light by his White sports agent played by Tom Cruise. In 2004, Morgan Freeman played Eddie Dupris, the supportive and encouraging older friend figure whose role is largely predicated upon ensuring that the White female lead character is cared for and supported in the attainment of her dreams.

In 2004 and 2006, Jamie Foxx and Forest Whitaker literally disappeared into their portrayals of the real life Ray Charles and Idi Amin, respectively. In *Ray,* Foxx portrayed the musical genius as both the embattled drug addict and womanizer history demonstrated him to be. In *The Last King of Scotland,* Whitaker's interpretation of the notorious Ugandan President Idi Amin's ruthlessness is chilling as he murders masses while acquiring great wealth for himself in a post-colonial Uganda. In Moonlight, Mahershala Ali portrays Juan, a crack dealer who provides a new perspective and a safe space for a teen navigating his life and sexuality as he grows toward manhood.

The SAG Awards are often seen as unique given that the honorees are selected and voted on by fellow artists. Many disciplines appreciate and support programs and systems of peer recognition. Although the winners of the SAG Awards often mirror the Oscars, they don't always. Since the inception of the award in 1994—first honorees awarded 1995—only four Black men have won for Outstanding Performance by a Male Actor in a Leading Role. The only non-duplicative win—when compared to the Oscar—in this category was Denzel Washington for his portrayal as Troy Maxson in the movie adaptation of August Wilson's *Fences.* Only five of the 24 men ever awarded the SAG award for Outstanding Performance by a Male Actor in a Supporting Role were Black. The only non-duplicative wins in this category were Eddie Murphy in *Dream Girls* (2006) and Idris Elba as The Commandant in *Beast of No Nations* (2015). Each of these actors, the stories they told, the narratives they interpreted and the characters they portrayed were valuable additions to the existing pool of work. The goal is to look at the roles that are created for these men and assess the nature of those that are celebrated by the industry's highest honors and not place blame on the men who did an outstanding job in their role. In each of these 12 instances (9 Oscar and 3 non-duplicative SAG), there are several patterns of over-represented themes and a striking absence of others.

The "magical negro" theme has long been discussed in film and television studies. Used as a narrative device, the Magical Negro is strategically placed in films and serves to teach White protagonists how to be better people, think: Uncle Remus, Oda Mae Brown, Bagger Vance and John Coffey. As it relates to the awarded characters, this theme is ever present in Eddie Dupris and Homer Smith who both arrive, miraculously save the day, help the White central characters meet their goals, facilitate their dreams and move the needle on their moral compasses. The magical negro often is either forced to ignore his own dreams to support those of the main characters or to make it appear that the two are aligned right before disappearing into the physical night of the evening or esoteric night of death.

The theme of the "Black Brute" is also over-represented in the celebration of these artists as characters like Alonzo Harris, Emil Foley, The Commandant and Idi Amin wield their hyper-masculinized and unscrupulous swords to literally and figuratively tear down other people, other Black people for the most part. Emil Foley's very first verbal assault in the film was on one of the only Black candidates in the initial line up played by Harold Sylvester. Alonzo Harris terrorizes an entire community under the shield of a police badge. When the attempts of his clean cut, White, rookie partner played by Ethan Hawke, to civilize him continue to fail, he is forced to expose him in a community brawl, saving this marginalized community of color from the sadistic Black police officer.

One may argue that characters like Idi Amin, The Commandant and Ray Charles were all actual people and if those stories are to be told, there is a need for Black actors to portray them. Although this is true, it is not the concern of note. These images in the absence of other celebrated images continue to support the disparate narratives of who Black men are. Certainly there are celebrated anti-social White male protagonists like the narcissistically abusive conductor Terrence Fletcher in *Whiplash* (2014) played by SAG award winner J.K. Simmons or the barbaric cannibal Dr. Hannibal Lecter in *The Silence of the Lambs* (1991) played by Academy Award winner Anthony Hopkins. In 1987s *Wall Street*, Michael Douglas was awarded for his portrayal of Gordon Gekko, an underhanded, heartless stock broker-turned corporate raider who didn't blink at tearing lives apart. Each of these roles supports anti-social imagery of White men in the same egregious ways described for the aforementioned Black character actors. Fortunately, however, for White men, they are celebrated and awarded far more often for pro-social roles than not.

Most people share fond memories of Tom Hanks' award-winning performances as Andrew Beckett, the beloved gay attorney who contracts AIDS in *Philadelphia* (1993) and Forest Gump (1994). Coln Firth's portrayal of King George VI in *The Kings Speech* (2010), Daniel Day-Lewis' work as Abraham Lincoln in *Lincoln* (2012) and Ed Harris' depiction of Gene Kranz in *Apollo 13* (1995) all provide a balance of imagery for White men in media that supports a heterogeneous view of their personhood and disproportionately situates them as heroes and saviors rather than brutes and thugs.

An additional layer of inquiry provides valuable information that completes the circle of this insidious narrative aimed to consistently highlight vilified Black maleness while negating Black male honorability, resilience and nobility. Looking at the anti-social roles for which these men were awarded is one thing, a look at the nominations for the pro-social roles that weren't celebrated during the dominant culture awards seasons provides additional clarity. In 1992, Denzel Washington was nominated for his transformative role as Malcolm X. In 2001, Will Smith was nominated for portraying Muhammed Ali. Malcolm X and Muhammed Ali were both self-assured, unapologetic civil rights leaders who ensured that disenfranchised Blacks were empowered and advocated for. In 2004, Don Cheadle was nominated for his role as Paul Rusesabagina in *Hotel Rwanda* where he worked to fight against genocide and save the lives of a multitude of people. In 2009, Morgan Freeman was nominated for his role as South African leader and world freedom icon Nelson Mandela in *Invictus*. None of these men won in their respective categories. Some might question the particular portrayal/performance, the script or the production as reasons these roles failed to garner the coveted prize. Some might say that Al Pacino's portrayal of Lt. Colonel Frank Slade in *Scent of a Woman* outshined Denzel as Malcolm X or that Jeff Bridges out-acted Morgan Freeman during their award cycle. For some, these explanations may ring true, but when contextualized, they appear to generate more questions than answers.

There have been many efforts to malign the characters of Black men across the globe. The author of *The Clansman*, Thomas F Dixon Jr. was born in 1864 in Shelby, NC, a small city near the western border of Charlotte. His father and grandfather owned enslaved Black Americans and were both members of the Ku Klux Klan (KKK). *The Clansman* was published in 1905, and one of its aims was to support the maintenance of systemic and institutionalized racial segregation across the nation through a siege of domestic terrorism. The perceived northern sympathy was a severe threat to the lucrative and oppressive systems of racism, Jim Crow and segregation saturating the American South.

In the same ways that television and film impact the imaging of Black men, so to do books and other forms of written communication. The KKK was founded in 1866 in Pulaski, TN, less than a full year after the institution of enslavement was abolished. Their objective was to fight against the Republican legislation aimed at increasing equity for Blacks after the Civil War. They wanted to maintain the oppression and suppression of Blacks, Jewish people, Catholics and others. The KKK created a campaign of hate imbedded in a system of fear and domestic terrorism. Their membership grew heartily but began to decline in the late 1800s until Dixon's publication provided the perfect vehicle to drive them back to prominence. Membership sky rocketed, partially due to adaptations of the book. The book was first adapted into a play, then a movie, *Birth of a Nation* (1915). This film, produced by D.W. Griffith and starring Lillian Gish, would catalyze the terrorism of the KKK and a movement against anyone who was not White Anglo-Saxon, Protestant and heterosexual. The KKK and other hate groups around the globe continue to grow stronger and stronger. Their efforts continue to gain more mainstream appeal and in some countries achieve a level of notable support in government election cycles.

In Conclusion

In today's ecosystem, we see the criminalization of Black male skin and bodies manifest itself in some of the most insidious ways. In an effort to ensure that Black people are blamed for their own victimization and oppression, ideologies of etiology are sensationalized to distract researchers and observers from the actual state of affairs. Constructs for which causal relationships are created between factors that are either non-unique to the Black community or those that actually provide evidence to support the existence of oppressive systems and not some mystical intrinsic mechanism of self-destruction are consistently highlighted.

The Bell Curve, by Charles Murray and Richard Herrnstein, was published in 1994 and uses evidence to suggest, again, that people of African descent are genetically inferior to other races and should be treated as such. The data presented in the text might bear some accuracy but the conclusions drawn from the data inspected were irresponsible and served to re-introduce the construct of IQ as a determining factor on experiences with and conditions of poverty, unemployment, crime and citizenship. They presented their arguments in a non-peer reviewed format to create a causal relationship between low IQ and undesirable and anti-social behavior including criminality, not voting in elections, school attrition and illegitimacy. The authors further indicated that the underpinning genetics of ethnicity played a role in innate cognitive abilities. The support of scientific racism and classism to justify disparate treatment against Blacks continues to maintain a system of inequity that bleeds into every facet of existence from child rearing and academic access to the literal factors that impact life and death outcomes (Hernstein & Murray, 1994).

Today, this research is coming back into the mainstream with individuals calling themselves "race realists", often publishing in journals like *Mindkind Quarterly*, created in the 1960s when their research was largely rejected by more traditional scientific journals. Its editor-in-chief, Gerhard Meisenberg, endorses biological differences in intelligences between racial groups, and its authors have been connected to racists' ideologies and White nationalist's organizations. Meisenberg and his assistant editor, Richard Lynn, have served on the editorial advisory boards for some highly regarded scientific publications (Saini, 2018). This paradigm continues into modern times. An investigation was launched in 2018 to determine how senior academic officials at the University College of London were able to host a series of secret conferences on eugenics and intelligence with speeches from noted White supremacists over a three-year period (Rawlinson & Adams, 2018).

The experiences of Black men are heavily impacted by public political violence and mass media vilification across the world. These factors feed an environment's ability to disenfranchise Black men in ways that negatively impact not only socio-cultural outcomes but behavioral health ones as well. This phenomenon is insidiously effective as it creates a damaging reciprocal relationship between the ecologies in which these men exist and the internal psychosocial risk factors that often inform outcomes for them and their progeny. Public political violence refers to the well-documented and exposed institutional forces and associated events that have legislated the systemic disenfranchisement of Black men and crystallized many maladaptive self-schemas that inform behavior, attitude and aptitude. Mass media vilification refers to the disproportionate promotion of images and caricatures that support stereotypical conceptualizations of failure, criminality, skewed masculinity and mental instability in Black men. The synergy between the two constructs worsens the obstacles Black men and boys face across the lifespan and contribute to the disproportionate burden of racialized stress.

References

Adiele, P. O. (2017). *The Popes, the Catholic Church and the Transatlantic Enslavement of Black Africans 1418–1839.* Hildesheim: Georg Olms Publishing.

Allen, K. (2018). *Hotel Employee Who Asked Black Guest to Leave Fired.* CNN. Retrieved from https://www.cnn.com/2018/12/28/us/portland-hotel-police-Black-guest-trnd/index.html

Amnesty International. (2011). *France: Our Lives Are Left Hanging France: Families of Victims of Deaths in Police Custody Wait for Justice to Be Done.* London: Amnesty International Publishing. Retrieved from https://www.amnesty.org/download/Documents/28000/eur210032011en.pdf

Arkansas Federal Writer's Project-Henry Blanks. US Work Project Administration. *History Matters.* Retrieve from http://historymatters.gmu.edu/d/6377/

Baptiste, E. (2015). *The Half Has Never Been Told: Slavery and the Making of Modern Capitalism.* New York: Basic Books.

BBC. (2015). *Mark Duggan Death: Timeline of Events.* Retrieved from https://www.bbc.com/news/uk-england-london-14842416

Beckert, S. (2014). *Empire of Cotton: A Global History.* New York: Alfred A. Knopf.

Bergman, J. (2014). *The Darwin Effect: Its Influence on Nazism, Eugenics, Racism, Communism.* Green Forest, AR: Capitalism & Sexism. Master Books.

Bernal, E. (2013). Rivers' Role: A Deeper Look Into Nurse Eunice Rivers Laurie. *The Tuskegee News.* Retrieved from http://www.thetuskegeenews.com/news/rivers-role-a-deeper-look-into-nurse-eunice-rivers-laurie/article_47f97284-7a37-5b4b-b2e9-9566570b4dae.html

Blackmon, D. (2008). *Slavery by Another Name: The Re-enslavement of Black Americans from the Civil War to World War II.* New York: Double Day.

Brown, D. (2017). A Surgeon Experimented on Slave Women Without Anesthesia. Now His Statues Are Under Attack. *The Washington Post.* Retrieved from https://www.washingtonpost.com/news/retropolis/wp/2017/08/29/a-surgeon-experimented-on-slave-women-without-anesthesia-now-his-statues-are-under-attack/?utm_term=.5e7f88cc631b

Canadian Broadcast Company (CBC). (2017). *Almost Half of TDSB Students Expelled Over Last 5 Years Are Black.* Report Says. Retrieved from https://www.cbc.ca/news/canada/toronto/almost-half-of-tdsb-students-expelled-over-last-5-years-are-Black-report-says-1.4065088

CBS News. (2018, July 18). *Bodies Exhumed from Unmasked Cemetery in Texas.* Retrieved from https://www.youtube.com/watch?v=jUznbz1YmrI

Chhor, K. (2016). *French Students Most Affected by Social Inequality, OECD Finds.* France 24. Retrieved from https://www.france24.com/en/20161207-french-students-most-affected-socioeconomic-disadvantages-oecd-pisa-study

City News. (2016). *Police Shooting of Jermaine Carby Began with Carding Officer Testifies.* Retrieved from https://toronto.citynews.ca/2016/05/12/fatal-police-shooting-of-jermaine-carby-began-with-carding-officer-testifies/

Clark, P. (1998). A Legacy of Mistrust: African-Americans, the Medical Profession, and AIDS. *The Linacre Quarterly, 65*(1), 66–88.

CNN. (2018). *Trayvon Martin Shooting Fast Facts.* CNN. Retrieved from https://www.cnn.com/2013/06/05/us/trayvon-martin-shooting-fast-facts/index.html

Commission on Systemic Racism in the Ontario Criminal Justice System. (1995). *Report.* Retrieved from http://www.ontla.on.ca/library/repository/mon/25005/185733.pdf

Coughlan, S. (2015). Study Reveals School Segregation. *BBC News.* Retrieved from https://www.bbc.com/news/education-33409111

Daniel, P. (1972). *We Are Going to Do Away with These Boys...* American Heritage. Retrieved from https://www.americanheritage.com/content/%E2%80%9Cwe-are-going-do-away-these-boys-%E2%80%A6%E2%80%9D

Davidson, E. (1997). *The Making of Adolf Hitler: The Birth and Rise of Nazism.* Columbia: University of Missouri Press.

Diallo, R. (2017). *Do Black Lives Matter in France?* Al Jazeera. Retrieved from https://www.aljazeera.com/indepth/opinion/2017/08/police-violence-france-justice-adama-170804091317713.html

DiManno, R. (2017). *Police Officer Who Shot Andrew Loku Describes the Last 21 Seconds of His Life.* The Star. Retrieved from https://www.thestar.com/news/gta/2017/06/14/police-officer-who-shot-andrew-loku-describes-the-last-21-seconds-of-his-life-dimanno.html

Domonoske, C., & Brown, T. (2018). *Milwaukee Police Disciplined for Using Stun Gun on, Arresting NBA Payer.* NPR. Retrieved from https://www.npr.org/sections/thetwo-way/2018/05/23/613657447/milwaukee-police-disciplined-for-tasing-arrest-of-nba-player

Draaisma, M. (2017). Black Students in Toronto Streamed Into Courses Below Their Ability, Reports Find. *CBC News.* Retrieved form https://www.cbc.ca/news/canada/toronto/study-Black-students-toronto-york-university-1.4082463

Fasick, K., & Steinbuch. (2015). Amadou Diallo's Furious Mom: Bratton Owes Me an Explanation. *New York Post.* Retrieved from https://nypost.com/2015/12/19/amadou-diallos-furious-mom-bratton-owes-me-an-explanation/

Finch, C. (1987). *The Black Roots of Egypt's Glory.* Washington Post. Retrieved from https://www.washingtonpost.com/archive/opinions/1987/10/11/the-Black-roots-of-egypts-glory/1c3faf74-331c-4cc1-a6a0-3535fa3e098a/?utm_term=.02841956d2c4

Franklin, J., & Moss, A. (1988). *From Slavery to Freedom: A History of Negro America.* New York: McGraw Hill.

Gillborn, D. (2008). Coincidence or Conspiracy? Whites, Policy and the Persistence of the Black/White Achievement Gap. *Education Review, 60*(3), 229–248.

Gillborn, D., Demack, S., Rollock, N., & Warmington, P. (2017). Moving the Goalposts: Education Policy and 25 Years of the Black/White Achievement Gap. *British Educational Research Journal, 43*(5), 848–874.

Gillis, W. (2015). *No Charges Against Peel Police in Death of Jermaine Carby*. The Star. Retrieved from https://www.thestar.com/news/crime/2015/07/21/no-charges-against-peel-police-in-death-of-jermaine-carby.html

Graber, H. (2017). *France's Ferguson*. Slate. Retrieved from https://slate.com/cover-stories/2017/01/the-death-of-adama-traore-has-become-frances-ferguson.html

Hallinan, M. (Ed.). (2000). *Handbook of the Sociology of Education*. New York: Springer.

Hamlin, C. (2018). *Videos Show Black Student in Handcuffs, Arrested for Wearing a Bandana in School*. Retrieved from https://newsone.com/3822540/Black-arizona-student-arrest-bandanna-videos/

Hansen, M., Levesque, E., Valant, J., & Quintero, D. (2018). *The 2018 Brown Center Report on American Education; How Well are American Students Learning?* Brown Center on Education Policy at Brookings. Retrieved from https://www.brookings.edu/wp-content/uploads/2018/06/2018-Brown-Center-Report-on-American-Education_FINAL.pdf

Held, A. (2018). *Men Arrested at Philadelphia Starbuck Speak Out: Police Commissioner Apologizes*. NPR. Retrieved from https://www.npr.org/sections/thetwo-way/2018/04/19/603917872/they-can-t-be-here-for-us-men-arrested-at-philadelphia-starbucks-speak-out

Hernstein, R., & Murray, C. (1994). *The Bell Curve: Intelligence and Class Structure in American Life*. New York: Free Press.

Historic Canada. *End of Segregation*. Retrieved from http://www.Blackhistorycanada.ca/events.php?themeid=7&id=9

Hohman, M. (2018). Parents of Black Wrestler Forced to Cut Dreadlocks Blame Referee Previously Accused of Using Slur. *People*. Retrieved form https://people.com/human-interest/family-Black-high-school-wrestler-cut-dreadlocks-speak/

Honjo, K. (2004). Social Epidemiology: Definition, History, and Research Examples. *Environmental Health and Preventive Medicine, 9*(5), 193–197.

Independent Office for Police Conduct. (2018). *Deaths During or Following Police Contact*. Statistics for England and Wales. Retrieved from https://www.police-conduct.gov.uk/sites/default/files/Documents/statistics/deaths_during_following_police_contact_201718.pdf

James, G. (1954). *Stolen Legacy: The Egyptian Origins of Western Philosophy*. Eastford, CT: Martino Fine Books.

Justia US Law. (1967). *Hobson v. Hansen, 269 F.* Supp. 401 (D.D.C. 1967). Retrieved from https://law.justia.com/cases/federal/district-courts/FSupp/269/401/1800940/

Kenney, T. (2018). *Memphis Teen Arrested for Violating Mall's 'No Hoodie' Policy, Black Man Detained for Defending Him.* Atlanta Black Star. Retrieved from https://atlantaBlackstar.com/2018/11/07/memphis-teen-arrested-for-violating-malls-no-hoodie-policy-Black-man-detained-for-defending-him/

Kirp, D. (2010). The Widest Achievement Gap. *National Affairs.*

Kitossa, T. (2018). *Tough Words in Toronto.* US News and World Report. Retrieved from https://www.usnews.com/news/cities/articles/2018-10-22/torontos-mayor-and-the-code-words-fueling-anti-Black-racism-in-canada

Larry, P. v Riles. NO C-71-2270 RFP. 495 F. Supp. 926. United States District Court, N. D. California.

Le Parisien. (2011). *Rally for Abu Bakari Tandia, Dead After Being Held in Police Custody.* Retrieved from http://www.leparisien.fr/hauts-de-seine-92/rassemblement-pour-abou-bakari-tandia-mort-apres-sa-garde-a-vue-24-01-2011-1240593.php

Leeuwen, A. (2018). The End of 'Zwarte Piet'? Jut Soot Pete's at Arrival of Sinterklaas in 2018. *The Dutch Review.* [Levelt]. Retrieved from https://dutchreview.com/culture/holidays/the-end-of-zwarte-piet-just-soot-petes-at-arrival-of-sinterklaas-in-2018/

Lepsius, R. (1853). *Letters from Egypt, Ethiopia, and the Peninsula of Sinai.* London: Henry G. Bohn.

Leslie, M. (2000). The Vexing Legacy of Lewis Terman. *Stanford Magazine.* Retrieved from https://stanfordmag.org/contents/the-vexing-legacy-of-lewis-terman

Levelt, S. (2018). *Do You Want Some Racism with Your Fries?* One World. Retrieved from https://www.oneworld.nl/mensenrechten/hoe-mcdonalds-deze-week-zwarte-piet-uitbande/

Little, B. (2018). *This Notorious Christmas Character is Dividing a Country.* National Geographic. Retrieved from https://news.nationalgeographic.com/2017/12/Black-pete-christmas-zwarte-piet-dutch/

Livingstone Smith, D. (2011). *Less Than Human: Why We Demean, Enslave, and Exterminate Others.* New York: St. Martins Press.

Lopez, G. (2018). *American Police Shoot and Kill Far More People Than Their Peers in Other Countries.* Vox. Retrieved from https://www.vox.com/identities/2016/8/13/17938170/us-police-shootings-gun-violence-homicides

Loveless, T. (2013). *The 2013 Brown Center Report on American Education: How Well Are American Students Learning.* Brookings Institute. Retrieved November 23, 2018, from https://www.brookings.edu/wp-content/uploads/2016/06/2013-brown-center-report-web-3.pdf

Lusane, C. (2002). *Hitler's Black Victims: The Historical Experiences of Afro-Germans, European Blacks, Africans, and African Americans in the Nazi Era.* London: Routledge.

Mansky, J. (2017). *P.T. Barnum Isn't the Hero the "Greatest Showman" Wants You to Think.* Smithsonian. Retrieved from https://www.smithsonianmag.com/history/true-story-pt-barnum-greatest-humbug-them-all-180967634/

Milner, J. T. (1890). *White Men of Alabama Stand Together: 1860 & 1890.* Birmingham, AL: McDavid Printing Company.

Murdoch, S. (2007). *IQ: A Smart History of a Failed Idea.* Hoboken, NJ: John Wiley & Sons, Inc.

Musson, A. E., & Robinson, E. (1969). *Science and Technology in the Industrial Revolution.* London: Gordon and Breach.

NAACP. (2016). *History of Lynchings.* Retrieved from https://www.naacp.org/history-of-lynchings/

Oduah, C. (2016). *The Afro-German Experience Under Hitler.* Huffington Post. Retrieved from https://www.huffingtonpost.com/chika-oduah/the-afroger-man-experience_b_9234700.html

Ogletree, C. (2010). *The Presumption of Guilt: The Arrest of Henry Louis Gates Jr. and Race, Class, and Crime in America.* New York: Palgrave Macmillan.

Ontario Human Rights Commission. (2017). Racial Profiling and Human Rights.14(1). Retrieved from http://www.ohrc.on.ca/sites/default/files/Racial%20Profiling%20and%20Human%20Rights_Canadian%20Diversity.pdf

Open Society Justice Initiative. (2009). *Profiling Minorities: A Study of Stop-and-Search Practices in Paris.* New York: Open Society Institute.

Pitts, T. (2005). Hugh M. Dorsey and "The Negro in Georgia". *The Georgia Historical Quarterly, 89*(2), 185–212.

Police Powers and Procedure England and Wales Statistics. (2018). *Ethnicity Facts and Figures: Race.* Retrieved from https://www.ethnicity-facts-figures.service.gov.uk/crime-justice-and-the-law/policing/number-of-arrests/latest

Rawlinson, K., & Adams, R. (2018). *UCL to Investigate Eugenics Conference Secretly Held on Campus.* The Guardian. Retrieved from https://www.theguardian.com/education/2018/jan/10/ucl-to-investigate-secret-eugenics-conference-held-on-campus

Rist, R. (1970). Social Class and Teacher Expectations: The Self-fulfilling Prophecy in Ghetto Education. *Harvard Educational Review, 40*(3), 411–451.

Ross, S. (2017). *AP Was There, Tuskegee Syphilis Study: Clinton Apologized.* Associated Press News. Retrieved from https://www.apnews.com/c10fe858b3384708aef94ad759c924f0

Saini, A. (2018). *Racism is Creeping Back Into Mainstream Science—We Have to Stop It.* The Guardian. Retrieved from https://www.theguardian.com/commentisfree/2018/jan/22/eugenics-racism-mainstream-science

Shiner, M., Carre, Z., Delsol, R., & Eastwood, N. (2018). *The Colour of Injustice: 'Race', Drugs and Law Enforcement in England and Wales.* Retrieved from http://www.stop-watch.org/uploads/documents/The_Colour_of_Injustice.pdf

Small Arms Survey. (2018). Retrieved from http://www.smallarmssurvey.org/de/about-us/highlights/2018/highlight-bp-firearms-holdings.html

Sotero, M. M. (2006). A Conceptual Model of Historical Trauma: Implications for Public Health Practice and Research. *Journal of Health Disparities Research and Practice, 1*(1), 93–108.

Strager, H. (2014). *A Modest Genius: The Story of Darwin's Life and How His Ideas Changed Everything.* Create Space Independent Publishing Platform.

Strand, S. (2012). The White British—Black Caribbean Achievement Gap: Tests, Tiers and Teacher Expectations. *British Educational Research Journal, 38*(1), 75–101.

Taylor, D. (2018). *Rashan Charles's Death After Police Chase Was Accident, Jury Finds.* The Guardian. Retrieved from https://www.theguardian.com/uk-news/2018/jun/20/rashan-charles-death-police-chase-was-accident-jury-finds

Terman, L. (1925). Genetic Studies of Genius. Mental and Physical Traits of a Thousand Gifted Children. Stanford, CA: Stanford University Press. Retrieved November 21, 2018, from https://archive.org/stream/geneticstudiesof009044mbp/geneticstudiesof009044mbp_djvu.txt

The Canadian Press. (2017). Officers Shot at Andrew Loku in 'Fear of Black Man with a Hammer,' Family's Lawyer Says. *CBC News.* Retrieved from https://www.cbc.ca/news/canada/toronto/loku-inquest-closing-arguments-1.4178077

The Challenge. (2017). *Understanding School Segregation in England: 2011–2016.* Retrieved from https://the-challenge.org/cms/uploads/page/policy-and-campaigns/tcn-understanding-school-segregation-in-england-2011-to-2016.pdf

The Challenge. *Research Reveals the Worrying Extent of Segregation in UK Schools.* Retrieved from https://the-challenge.org/five-minutes/research-reveals-the-worrying-extent-of-segregation-in-uk-schools/

The Global Burden of Disease 2016 Injury Collaborators. Global Mortality from Firearms, 1990–2016. *JAMA.*

The Guardian. (2015). *Mark Duggan Shooting: Armed Officers Charged of Wrongdoing.* Retrieved from https://www.theguardian.com/uk-news/2015/mar/25/armed-police-cleared-wrongdoing-fatal-shooting-mark-duggan-tottenham

The Opportunity Agenda. *Media Portrayals and Black Male Outcomes.* Retrieved from https://opportunityagenda.org/explore/resources-publications/media-representations-impact-Black-men/media-portrayals

The Tuskegee Experiment. (2015). *Eunice Rivers: Friend or Foe?* Retrieved from http://tuskegeesyphilis.weebly.com/blog/eunice-rivers-friend-or-foe

Turda, M., & Weindling, P. (Eds.). (2007). *Blood and Homeland: Eugenics and Racial Nationalism in Central and Southeast Europe 1900–1940.* Budapest: Central European University Press.

US Const. amend. XIII, sec. 1

Wall, L. L. (2006). The Medical Ethics of Dr J Marion Sims: A Fresh Look at the Historical Record. *Journal of Medical Ethics, 32*(6), 346–350.

Washington, H. (2006). *Medical Apartheid: The Dark History of Medical Experimentation on Black Americans from Colonial Times to the Present.* New York: Harlem Moon.

Weld, D. T. (1839). *American Slavery As It Is: Testimony of a Thousand Witnesses.* New York: Dover Publications.

Wikipedia. *Academy Award for Best Actor.* Retrieved from https://en.wikipedia.org/wiki/Academy_Award_for_Best_Actor

Wikipedia. *Screen Actors Guild Award for Outstanding Performance by a Male Actor in a Leading Role.* Retrieved from https://en.wikipedia.org/wiki/Screen_Actors_Guild_Award_for_Outstanding_Performance_by_a_Male_Actor_in_a_Leading_Role

Williams, G. (2010). *Angel of Death; The Story of Smallpox.* New York: Palgrave Macmillan.

Willsher, K. (2018). *Police Officer Arrested Over Shooting That Sparked Nantes Riots.* The Guardian. Retrieved from https://www.theguardian.com/world/2018/jul/05/security-forces-dispatched-to-nantes-after-police-shooting-sparks-violence

Winfield, A. (2007). *Eugenics and Education in America: Institutionalized Racism and the Implications of History, Ideology, and Memory.* New York: Peter Lang.

Wolters, R. (2008). *Race and Education 1954–2007.* Columbia: University of Missouri Press.

CHAPTER 6

Noose Knots: *Data Paralysis and Oppressive Psychological Tactics*

Equifinality is a concept that describes a flexibility of response within an open system—biological and social—that explains how several paths lead to the same destination. When discussing agriculture, evolution, mental illness or behaviors like philanthropy or intimate partner violence, research demonstrates that there are several ways in which individuals and systems have reached the status at which they exist when we engage them. Systems theory emphasizes the interactive structures and modules in which people exist and uses equifinalty to value the varied roads that lead to the same destinations. Systems and the individuals in them acquire tools and attributes through the experiential learning process born from life's varied interactions and experiences. This process results in a simultaneous cycle of continued evolution for both the system and the individual across the lifespan (Mills, Durepos, & Wiebe, 2010).

Contemporary outcomes for Black men across a nation influence and are influenced by the environmental containers in which they develop. These containers hold historical and contemporary events, ancestors of the immediate and ancient pasts, living family and community members in addition to the general systemic actors and observers. The Greek philosopher Aristotle wrote "It is thus clear that, just as some are by nature free, so others are by nature slaves, and for these latter, the condition of slavery is both beneficial and just". Although Aristotle didn't label these "others" as sub-human, he did implicate a perceived "rudimentary" ability to reason as a characteristic that rendered them human-like, but certainly not

© The Author(s) 2019
D. E. Grant Jr., *Black Men, Intergenerational Colonialism, and Behavioral Health*, https://doi.org/10.1007/978-3-030-21114-1_6

human. Greek culture saw themselves as the innovators and intellects of the world during their time and referenced all others as "barbaroi" or barbarians, unable to effectively reason with depth, reflection or intentionality (Livingstone Smith, 2011).

When one controls for geographic location and socio-economic status, the world sees a wide variety of similar outcomes for Black men across the diaspora. Experiences and conditions like unemployment, poverty, substance abuse, school attrition, mortality for non-fatal conditions and incarceration are more common among Black men when compared to other men in similar ecological strata. As boys, some of these men lived in homes with married parents while others never knew one of their parents. Some of these men attended college while others never finished high school. Some come from a history of physical and sexual abuse while others consistently developed under the watchful protection of trusted caregivers. Every Black boy is born with the capacity to achieve success, great success. The open systems into which they are born, like equifinality describes, is riddled with a multitude of risk factors that often render them in disproportionate danger to the oppressive devices of their fellow human being, no matter where or how their journey began.

A January 1928 issue of the British "Anti-Slavery Monthly Reporter" quoted the reflections of Roman senator and historian Tacitus:

> … (T) here is nothing so sweet to the human heart, as the gratification which arises from the consciousness of having the life of a fellow-creature at one's disposal. And it is this prevailing love of power which presents, perhaps, the greatest obstacle to the abolition of slavery … Power in the hands of men, is in no instance so much subject to abuse, as in its exercise over their own species. (The Anti-Slavery Monthly, 1828, p. 2)

Based on the worldviews and practices associated with European imperialism, it would appear that the paradigms of Aristotle and other Greeks were very influential. Those who participated, authorized and profited from the institution of imperialism and the associated practices must have certainly been familiarized with his work, particularly given the alignment of behaviors and viewpoints. Information on the literacy rates of European imperialists and their immediate ancestors is conflicting at best. Research identifies variables like country, geography within the country, wealth, gender, socio-cultural role and language of origin as factors in the disparate statistics on European literacy during and preceding the Transatlantic Slave Trade. As a result, it is difficult to ascertain the precise influence that

Greek writings on slavery and oppression had on the cultural paradigms of common Europeans and colonial planters of the time. It is, however, relatively clear that the tools, strategies and practices align strongly with those philosophies.

Colonialism is often inappropriately thought of in a single context, confined to a single space and time. Several constructs have been identified that render the legacy of colonialism and enslavement alive and well in contemporary times. Bulhan (2015) describes the effects that colonialism has had on the contemporary ecosystem by illustrating the sustained "Eurocentric epistemology, ontology, and ideology emanating from, supporting, and validating (the) European monopoly of power" that held supremacy over the nations that were colonized. These systems also defined the status quo for Euronormative nations where men of African descent exist. These phenomena represent a value system that extends beyond the acute events of colonization. Coloniality and metacolonialism are often used interchangeably throughout research. Unlike colonialism, coloniality "denotes enduring patterns of power as well as a way of thinking and behaving that emerged from colonialism but survived long after its seeming demise" (Bulhan, 2015). Written history often highlights the benevolent colonists and the savages being colonized, all contextualized in a contemporary environment where the oppressive forces continue to set forth the normative attributes of the societies that dominate the subordinate.

Quijano and Ennis (2000) describe the codification of race, operationalized in the genotype's melanin production, as a basis for subjugation. As a result, "the conquered and dominated peoples were situated in a natural position of inferiority" (Quijano & Ennis, 2000) as were their physical features, intellectual capabilities and cultural traditions. In a 1969 issue of the Harvard Review, psychologist Arthur Jensen published *How Much Can We Boost IQ and Scholastic Achievement?* In this paper, Dr. Jensen made several conclusions based on his research, including the failure of Head Start Programs to demonstrate increases in IQ scores for Black children as it had been partially intended. Dr. Jensen stated that this failure was because 80% of intellectual variance was reliant on genetic qualities for Black students, leaving only 20% for environmental efforts, like Head Start, parent engagement activities and other social programs. Dr. Jensen's work further stated that these factors were unchangeable because general cognitive ability was an inherited trait.

By the 1970s, hundreds of Black American boys had been funneled into special education classes and day schools. They had been labeled as "mentally retarded" and cognitively flawed as a direct result of Binet's tests of intelligence, those tests developed upon the same foundation and the crystallized belief of the hereditarian theory. This became so much of a problem that in 1979, US District Judge Robert F. Peckham barred public schools in the state of California from using standardized IQ tests to determine whether or not Black children should be placed in special education classes because the tests were "racially and culturally biased" (Wyatt et al., 2003). It was clear at this time that these practices of inequity not only created false labels but also led to dead-end programs of under-education for Black boys resulting in intergenerational under-employment and disproportionate poverty (Merl, 1991). The following is the ruling made by the California court:

> The court finds in favor of plaintiffs, the class of Black children who have been or in the future will be wrongly placed or maintained in special classes for the educable mentally retarded (EMR). On plaintiffs' statutory and state and federal constitutional claims. In violation of Title VI of the Civil Rights Act of 1964, the Rehabilitation Act of 1973, and the Education for All Handicapped Children Act of 1975, defendants have utilized standardized intelligence tests that are racially and culturally biased, have a discriminatory impact against Black children, and have not been validated for the purposes of essentially permanent placements of Black children into educationally dead-end, isolated,and stigmatizing classes for the so-called educable mentally retarded. Further, these federal laws have been violated by defendants' general use of placement mechanisms that, taken together, have not been validated and result in a large overrepresentation of Black children in the special and EMR classes. (Larry P. v Riles, NO C-71-2270 RFP. 495 F. Supp. 926)

In spite of rulings like this, discussions and publications on Black intellectual inferiority continued the maintenance of this paradigm into the twenty-first century. In 1994, Richard Herenstein and Charles Murray published "The Bell Curve" which further indicted genetic inferiority for the performance of Black children across most domains of intelligence. This 800-page book sold hundreds of thousands of copies around the world and was translated into many different languages. Other twentieth- and twenty-first-century books that promote biogenetic inferiority include: *Why Race Matters* (1997) by Michael Levin, *The g Factor* (1998) by Arthur

Jenson and *TABOO: Why Black Athletes Dominate: Sports and Why We Are Afraid to Talk About It* (2001) by Jon Entine.

When put together, these philosophies and publications contribute to a system of education, from Head Start and kindergarten through high school and college. They birth practices that implicitly and explicitly track dispro-portionate numbers of Black boys into domains of adult peril. The School to Prison Pipeline represents one of these systems where the final destina-tion for many Black boys is incarceration and/or interment. Constructs like Learned Helplessness, Stereotype Threat and Self-Fulfilling Prophecy oper-ationalize themselves in the world as high drop-out rates, dismal graduate degree attainment and a prison industrial complex filled with men of color.

There is a regular discussion that occurs related to the numbers of Black men in college versus those who are either incarcerated or under some cur-rent state or federal supervision as a result of parole or probation. In one 2013 article, Dr. Ivory A. Toldson, Editor-in-Chief of the Journal for Negro Education and former Executive Director of President Obama's White House initiative on HBCU's, asks what the line "There are more Black men in jail than in college" has in common with the Jheri curl. Answer: "They were invented by White men ... and adopted enthusiasti-cally by Black people, and they left a nasty stain on the shoulders of mil-lions of Black men" (Scharff et al., 2010). In 2000, a Justice Policy Institute report entitled *Cellblocks or Classroom: The Funding of Higher Education and Corrections and Its Impact on African American Men* indicated that in the year 2000, there were 791,600 Black men under the jurisdiction of a federal, state or local penal system compared to 603,032 enrolled in insti-tutions of higher education (Justice Policy Institute, 2002). The authors wrote, "A third more African American men are incarcerated than in higher education". The American Council on Education demonstrates that after 2002, data collection practices were adjusted to address the age strata to include both groups stage of eligibility more deliberately, to include schools that had not participated in past surveys, and students who registered after the Fall semester (American Council on Education, 2012). Each of these factors held responsibility for the irresponsible under-estimation of Black male matriculation in years prior to 2002. Raw data demonstrated that from 2001 to 2013, Black male college enrollment grew by 107% from 693,044 to 1,437,363 (Desmond-Harris, 2015). The importance in addressing this myth is multi-faceted, and Dr. Toldson explains why acade-micians must work to let the complete data set tell the story. He explains that this myth promotes a system that fails to adequately attend to the Black male academics by implying that they don't exist and where they do, the numbers are too miniscule to dedicate resources and programming. Black male academics are, as a result, rendered invisible (Desmond-Harris, 2015). It is important to note that in dismantling this myth, it is still important to attend to the issues with Black male over-incarceration.

TEACHING HELPLESSNESS

Learned Helplessness is a theory grounded in the notion that all animals including humans can learn the uncontrollability of reinforcers. In situations labeled "uncontrollable", the probability that a behavior will elicit a particular outcome is equal to that outcome's presence in the absence of the same behavior. People feel out of control when making decisions given that both action and inaction are met with the same outcome. Marginalized groups experience this uncontrollability with a higher degree of frequency when compared to their peers of dominant culture. As a result, they are more susceptible to and disproportionately represented among those with cognitive deficits, lowered self-esteem, depressed mood or who procrastinate, give up prematurely and exhibit an inhibition of behavioral responses and other concerns associated with learned helplessness (Hockenbury & Hockenbury, 2004; Kenyon, 1994; Thomas, 1986).

Perceived or actual uncontrollability leading to learned helplessness has been identified as most prevalent in certain environments and systems. Individuals who experience incarceration, war, disability, marginalization and/or poverty are exposed to increased opportunities to experience the type of uncontrollability that lends itself to learned helplessness. Uncontrollability is usually conceptualized by those who perceive/experience it in three primary ways: personal, pervasive or permanent. Individuals who conceptualize uncontrollability as personal tend to internalize negative life events and see themselves as the problem and primary success obstacle. Giving up prematurely becomes easy when this paradigm is adopted, particularly as many marginalized individuals are rarely instilled with the belief that they have the tools to fix themselves. Many of these individuals hold the belief that an innate lack of ability creates and sustains their problems, a major step on the route toward the crystallization of both helplessness and hopelessness, a dangerous combination. Individuals who conceptualize uncontrollability as pervasive and/or permanent believe that their perceived uncontrollability will exist in all areas of their life forever. The hopelessness associated with both these paradigms renders people unable to move as it is presupposed that all activity will result in failure in every domain and that time is not likely to change that.

The negative outcomes and deficits associated with learned helplessness are also divided into three domains: motivational, cognitive and emotional (Kenyon, 1994). Individuals experiencing the motivational deficits associated with learned helplessness may not try and influence change into their own situation. Their helpless existentialism drains them of their desire to take action on goals or identified objectives. For those experiencing the negative cognitive outcomes of learned helplessness, a lack of skills and tools aimed at altering the helplessness of their circumstance(s) or condition(s) is one of the most striking characteristics. Finally, individuals suffering from the emotional injuries of learned helplessness might be depressed over their failure or inability to exert control over significant facets of their lives.

> Learned helplessness has detrimental effects on children. They develop a lack of self-confidence in challenging tasks which results in deterioration of performances. These children also use poor problem solving strategies; their attention wanders and they feel that they are struggling for nothing. This might even put learned helpless children behind a grade or two in academic subjects and damper their social skills. In the end, they get a message that they are worthless and hopeless. They feel incompetent and unable to master any new material or task. Learned helpless children "know" that they are failures and will not think otherwise. In Erikson's view, he suggests that children with few successes will become inferior which leads them to have a low self-esteem. Most learned helpless students give up trying to gain respect through their academic performance so they turn to other means for recognition. They may become the class clown, bully or tease. When they begin adolescent years they try to gain respect through antisocial behaviors. (Shields, 1997, p. 1)

Disidentification is the realignment of one's self-concept and values so that one's self-worth and esteem are no longer dependent on performance in a chosen environment. One might disidentify in order to relieve the pain of failure in arenas where success is unlikely. Failure can be painful, especially for male children who are beginning to interpret the messages their worlds and communities send them about themselves and their masculinity. In order to avoid that pain, it is posited that many of these boys convince themselves that school and education are not important facets of their world. This distortion is then validated in their environment as many of their peers disidentify with academia creating a dangerously maladaptive homogeneity of thought. Entire peer groups might be experiencing the same phenomenon with an equitably distributed set of ineffective tools to provide any viable alternatives. In many cases, disidentification is shaped and supported by negative teacher expectations, systems of academic tracking and limited teacher resource and supports (Honora, 2003).

Drs. Claude and Shelby Steele, twin brothers born on New Year's day in 1946 in Chicago, would both make important contributions to America. They come from working class roots, where their mother was a social worker with the Congress of Racial Equality (CORE) and their father a truck driver. These two men who shared a womb also share their thirst for higher education, for research and for discourse on marginalized communities. Where they diverge, and diverge sharply, is the nature of their research lens and the types of discourse in which they engage regarding these marginalized communities. Each one had a different view of the underlying community needs and the etiology of those needs. Dr. Shelby Steele is a noted Black conservative who has historically rallied against social programming that addresses injustice and equity issues. In 2007, he published *A Bound Man: Why We Are Excited about Obama and Why He Can't Win*, a book about the former US President's identity as a bi-racial, multi-cultural man being rigidly bound to what Steele described as a "Black identity" bundled with his politic. Dr. Claude Steele, through his research on stereotype threat, approached the concerns of the marginalized in a very different way.

Steele (1997) defined stereotype threat as an "apprehension over possibly self-fulfilling negative stereotypes about one's group, or being judged". In 1995, along with researcher Dr. Joshua Aronson, Steele conducted standardized test sessions that normalized the design to control for race expectation and preconception. Their results indicated that when presented with a test intended to assess ability, Black students performed dramatically worse than White students. When this same test was administered to a different set of similar students and framed as a problem solving task instead of a test of ability, Black student performance matched that of equally yoked White students. This valence change sent a message to the Black participants that the racial stereotype about their ability was irrelevant to performance on this task. This change extinguished what the researchers called the "stereotype spotlight". Researchers, across the years, have generalized this phenomenon to other populations across the content of varied "stereotype spotlights" including but not limited to: women taking math and science tests, older adults engaging in memory exercises and White male athletes being tested on natural athletic ability.

A 2004 study (Croizet, Depres, & Gauzins, 2004) of stereotype threat indicated that when individuals targeted by allegations of inferiority are placed into situations where this inferiority can be displayed, performance suffers. It suffers as a result of the extra cognitive and emotional load generated by the fear of fulfilling the allegations of inferiority presented by the stereotype. This study of 164 college students was the first to measure changes in mental workloads using one's "psychophysiological state" as gathered from non-intrusive neurological somatic response measurements. The data generated from this study supported Steele's earlier work and found that "test instructions that mention intellectual ability have a disruptive effect on the performance of people targeted by a reputation of lower intelligence. Under such conditions their performance drops and they underachieve in comparison to their peers" (Croizet et al., 2004, p. 728). When this same assessment is given without reference to intellectual ability, the stereotyped group shows improved performance.

A depletion in the capacity of working memory and impairments in knowledge acquisition are implicated as mechanisms by which stereotype threat produces some of the performance and social deficits experienced when confronted with the threat of supporting the stereotype (Grand, 2016). For many students, self-esteem has consistently had a direct relationship with academic performance. Research indicates that this is not always the case with Black students. "Disidentification relieves the pain of stereotype threat by breaking identification with the part of life where pain occurs, which necessarily includes a loss of motivation to succeed in (that) part of life ..." (Crosby & Van de Veer, 2000, p. 130). National Centers of Education Statistics (NCES) indicates a similar level of school achievement for all children regardless of race and gender up to the third and fourth grades, after which a downward trend begins with most all male students. While male students of other ethnicities tend to show improvement in achievement levels during middle school, the achievement rates of both Black and Hispanic boys continue to decline.

In 2011, *The Other Wes Moore: One Name, Two Fates* became one of the New York Times best-selling books, remaining on the list for over 40 weeks. While studying abroad during his senior year at Johns' Hopkins, the author—Wes Moore—learns about the tragic murder of Sgt Bruce Prothero—Baltimore County police sergeant, husband and father of five. He also learns about the man hunt for his murderer, Wes Moore. The book is a narrative of two men, both named Wes Moore, born blocks from one another in Baltimore. Each had strikingly similar backgrounds. They both came from working class families where poverty loomed near. They were both raised by single moms. The author's dad died when he was a child while the other never knew his. Both men of similar ages even had academic and disciplinary problems growing up. Given all these common-alities, how does one become a Rhodes scholar and the other a convicted murderer serving life in prison?

Self-fulfilling prophecy also known as the Rosenthal Effect is a phe-nomenon that demonstrates how one's expectations of another person actually affect the person's performance in measurable ways. Robert Rosenthal and Lenore Jacobson showed that teacher expectations of youth giftedness actually made a difference in learning gains as shown by scores on pre- and post-IQ tests. The researchers told the teachers that a random smattering of about 20% of their students were "intellectual bloomers" who could be expected to outperform the other students. As you might suspect, by the end of the study, the scores of all the children had improved, but the scores of each kid in the experimental group had improved in a statistically significant manner that differed from those of the control group (Rosenthal & Jacobson, 1966).

The Pygmalion and Golem Effect are corollary to one another. Where the former describes how people internalize their positive labels and grow pro-socially as a result, the latter demonstrates how low expectations lead to poorer performance. The story of the two Wes Moore's provides us with a great example of how people live up or down to the expectations set for them. Toward the end of the book, when the author asks the incar-cerated Moore if he believes that people are products of their environ-ments, he states that people's fates are determined by other people's expectations; if they are expected to succeed, they will succeed, and if they are expected to fail, they'll fail.

Together each of these factors—learned helplessness, stereotype threat, self-fulfilling prophecy—and their associated risks create complex ecosys-tems where Black men and boys live. They are positioned into situations where internal and external hazards increase their propensities to reside in spaces of dis-ease. Many people see this as a referendum to abscond Black men, their families and their communities from any personal accountabil-ity for their contemporary conditions when in fact, it is quite the contrary. When communities are able to understand the interconnectedness of sys-tems that create conditions, they and the systems are better equipped to advocate for a more responsible set of interventions that bring about authentic change. For instance, when we discuss intimate partner violence (IPV), practitioners, funding and programming are primarily aimed at support for survivors. This is a great need not to be ignored, but our dis-parate lack of attention to the exploration of a perpetrator's under-lying needs minimizes the system's ability to effect true change in this area. Many run away from the question "Why do men hit women?", because they are always confronted with "Well, a man should never hit a woman", and the discourse ends there. Until increased attention is paid to the models of developmental hyper-masculinity and global misogyny that contribute to male inadequacies and inabilities to manage anger, impulse, subordination and frustration in prosocial ways, violence against women will continue. These constructs are not presented to burden survivors of IPV or the systems in which they exist with blame, but to empower individuals, families, communities and systems to adopt a more holistic view of the issue to create intervention strategies that align with the scope and complexity of the concerns and conditions.

When assessing the scale and scope of the complex intersections of health and wellness for men of African descent across the diaspora, a very intricate portrait appears on the canvas. If it were a strength-based word map, it would include words to describe characteristics like resilience, healing, tender masculinity and post-traumatic growth. John Biggers, born in Gastonia, NC, just 60 years after slavery was abolished, is a noted Black American muralist. His murals, inspired by the Black American quilting tradition of the south and Mexican American muralists like Diego Rivera, held consistent messages forcing dialogue on ecological systems that work together to influence outcomes for Black families. His work often held multi-layered symbolism embedded in the painting's quilt-like sections and layers. In *Upper Room* (1983), he depicts two women carrying an edifice of some sort on their backs. To the left of these women is another woman—leaning on them for support—while co-facilitating the ascension of what appears to be two youth whose destination seems bound only by the capacity of the system to support their trajectory.

The analysis of systems from this lens provides an opportunity to ensure that we account for the ecosystem's participation in the outcomes we see for Black men living in Euronormative nations. The desire and right to grow to one's full potential should not have to be earned, yet we see a bargaining system between Black men and each of their nations to simply recognize (and hopefully acknowledge) their general humanity. The consistent impact of stress and stressors from: passive and active service denial, behaviors and motives of stigma-perpetuating structures, disproportionate epidemiology and morbidity of disease, and practices in mental health systems jeopardize Black male wellness.

One common theme concomitant with each salient feature is the individual and network stress loads that impact them in measurable and immeasurable ways. Research regarding stress and Black men consistently discusses the impact of unique psychological and socio-cultural stressors on their development across the lifespan. The American Psychological Association defines stress as "any uncomfortable emotional experience accompanied by predictable biochemical, physiological and behavioral changes" (American Psychological Association [APA]). The secretion of cortisol in the body is a function resulting from the activation of three interactive bodily regions: the brain's hypothalamus, and the body's pituitary and adrenal glands. These regions collectively make up the hypothalamic–pituitary–adrenal (HPA) axis. The HPA is activated when individuals are exposed to stress-inducing stimuli resulting in the production of cortisol. Some people describe cortisol as our internal security and fire alarm system.

Produced by adrenal glands, cortisol is a steroid hormone that is most famous for fueling the human "fight or flight" response. In order to effectively manage this anthropological response, cortisol also has access to and influence over the body's use of chemicals like proteins, fats and carbohydrates as well as functions like blood pressure regulation, memory formation, sleep and wake cycles and the production of energy for the management of stress. One consequence of cortisol's wide reach is the impact it has on overall health. Individuals who experience chronic stress are susceptible to somatic conditions due to the over use of the body's internal alarm system. Research demonstrates that health problems like anxiety, depression, heart disease, weight gain and memory problems might ensue as a result of chronic stress experiences that increase body functions' access to cortisol exposure (APA; Russell, Koren, Rieder, & Van Uum, 2014).

The practice of collecting cortisol from human subjects for the purposes of research on stress and overall health is well established. Cortisol is naturally secreted from the body through several very distinct bodily fluids, all associated with specific body functioning. The urine, perspiration, tears and blood of most all human beings have measurable sums of cortisol dissolved within them. Much of the research on cortisol composition has focused on testing these fluids to assess individual's levels of exposure to stressful stimuli. When compared to one another, different fluid samples taken from the same participants tended to contain comparable levels of cortisol (Russell et al., 2014). Although measurements of cortisol levels across fluid types demonstrated a high level of intraparticipant reliability, they were limited to measurements of acute levels of cortisol secretion, from as short as minutes to hours at most.

Stress indeed has an adaptive quality that promotes healthy growth and development, and as a result, everyone secretes its primary accompaniment, cortisol. Anxiety, insomnia, heart disease, obesity, depression and high blood pressure are just some of the conditions, diseases and disorders that are correlated to stress experiences. The myriad of health concerns that science has linked to stress exposure are not usually associated with acute stress, they are more often the responses to worry, pressure and strain suffered over a prolonged period of time known as chronic stress (Abell et al., 2016; APA).

In addition to bodily fluids, cortisol tends to secrete onto the hair follicles both directly and through the act of perspiration creating deposits over time, making it a biomarker for chronic stress. Although factors like deposits from perspiration, chemical processing and hair maintenance products all present uncontrollable variables for these studies, the outcomes remain noteworthy within the scope and depth of this particular study. Researchers (Abell et al., 2016) studied the hair cortisol concentration (HCC) of "British civil servants" most of whose last known civil service employment grade was at or above the level of "executive". The researchers found that the Black study participants had a higher concentration of cortisol in their hair samples when compared to other ethnic groups. Their concentrations were on average about 200% more than British South Asians and British Whites (Abell et al., 2016). A 2013 study published in Therapeutic Drug Monitoring looked at cortisol deposits in the hair of Canadian First Nations communities who experience higher incidences of chronic diseases, socio-economic disparity and cultural oppression when compared to their White Canadian counterparts. The researchers found that the average HCC in this group was "significantly higher" than the White control group (Henley et al., 2013). Although the need for more research on the biological markers of chronic stress remains relevant, these and other studies demonstrate strong evidence that certain groups provide physical confirmation of the disproportionate existence of chronic stress across the lifespan.

Stigma is defined as "the process whereby labelling, stereotyping, separation, status loss and discrimination occur together, often simultaneously in the context of power" (Mantovani, Pizzolati, & Edge, 2017, p. 374) to create or maintain systems that are dependent upon the stigma's resultant narrative. Euronormative nations have dedicated countless hours of cognitive energy and financial resources to the systematic labeling and creative stereotyping of Black men to develop a supportive narrative that would be sustained by formal separation. Due to segregation's propensity to provoke discrimination and a tangible elimination of contact points across races, Black men suffered severe position forfeiture. This penalization has painted the post-civil rights narrative which articulates the contemporary Black stigma. Each of those interconnected factors is known to promote the devaluation, rejection and exclusion of entire cohorts of people. It can often render them alone to deal with the stigmas that present themselves as social disadvantage and status decay. Stigma exists across three interactive levels—Social, Self and Structural—each of which reinforces the other.

The responses of industrialized nations to waves of mass drug addiction provide some of the most efficient vehicles through which to understand stigma and its mechanistic range. The loving and empathic responses from the world to the twenty-first-century North American opioid epidemic and its addict juxtaposed to the criminalization of the twentieth-century North American crack epidemic and its addict paints an intriguing picture of how stigma operationalizes itself in an open system. Social-stigma exists in spaces and contexts where dominant group members are conditioned to differentiate themselves from those who hold a set of devalued attributes. The characteristics under attack might be associated with race, medical condition, affectional orientation, mental illness or an intersection of them all.

Social stigma occurs when behaviors and attitudes of the dominant (non-target, oppressor) group publicly and privately endorse negative stereotypes, propaganda and oppressive legislation toward the non-dominant (target, oppressed) group. These endorsements also work to reinforce self and structural stigma as was seen with the crack cocaine epidemic of the 1980s and 1990s. In the early 1980s, drug dealers began to convert a bottle necked surplus of powdered cocaine into a solid form called crack that was cheaper, easier to move and meant to be smoked instead of snorted. Crack cocaine had existed since the 1970s but was popularized to epidemic proportions when officials of the US government passively allowed the product to saturate poor racialized communities in some of America's largest cities. By the mid-1980s, crack could be found in the urban areas of major cities across the USA, Canada and the Caribbean. The victims of this epidemic were largely poor people of color (Frontlines, PBS).

Casting the characteristic drug addict in White-dominated societies has been an intricately woven effort across national histories. Three centuries drenched with messaging aimed at crystallizing stigma to dependably "other" Black men and boys while mitigating damage to dominant culture perceptions of self has successfully created a set of steadfast stigma patterns that continue to disenfranchise Black men. America has seen a variety of philosophies related to how it treats substance abusers, the social capital ascribed to certain substances, the federal government scheduling of substances, the adjudication of abusers and the rehabilitation paradigms across chronosystems. Both Presidents Richard Nixon and Ronald Reagan adopted the philosophies that not only criminalized drugs, but created focused efforts to eradicate their abusers. The 1986 Anti-Drug Abuse law supported a zero-tolerance philosophy toward substance abusers and created mandatory sentencing for the distribution and possession of crack cocaine specifically. Crack cocaine was criminalized at a rate 100 times that of powder cocaine. Based on Congressional Record, this disparate criminalization ratio appears to be more arbitrary than not (Frontlines, PBS).

Research demonstrates that dominant culture promulgation of stereotypes works to catalyze and synergize existing environmental risk factors for individuals who endorse membership in one or more of the marginalized groups. Although Blacks represented fewer than 40% of crack users at the time, they represented over 80% of individuals convicted for crack possession and almost 90% of those convicted of trafficking. In 1995, the US Sentencing Commission indicated a need to address these disparities, but both Congress and President Bill Clinton failed to act upon the recommendation and the agreed upon dispensability of the Black crack addict resulted in another mass assault to the Black community and its future generations (Frontlines, PBS).

Once the social-stigma is firmly applied, the tried and true system relies upon itself to autonomously create—within the person, toward themselves—the same shame that social stigma introduced for the world's exploitation. Self-stigma occurs in individuals who hold group memberships that possess stigmatized attributes. These individuals are often socialized to believe that they and their existences are less valuable than that of others. Self-stigma not only negatively impacts service access and utilization, it also contributes to the adoption of feelings like shame and guilt that create anxiety associated with being identified as a member of the group for which the stigma is present. This continues to operationalize itself in one of the most insidious of the system's components, the one that renders intraracial engagements and fraternal supports fractured between Black men in a position to help and Black men positioned to be helped.

This self-stigma is usually supported by interactions with people of dominant culture who reinforce the stigma narrative through the exhibition of implicit and explicit actions that might vilify, ignore and/or trigger people of non-dominant groups. Individuals of the non-dominant groups often hold sufficient anecdotal and experiential data to attribute this treatment to their group membership (ethnicity, mental wellness status, affectional orientation). The true risk of self-stigma is the internalization of the feelings that result in negative self-image, reduced self-efficacy and a propensity to adopt intraculturally oppressive attitudes (self-hate) and the associated behaviors.

Structural bias often occurs as a result of social stigma's capacity to aggregate individuals, often professionals, into one space where they are charged with the care, service provision or support for individualized in stigmatized groups. This structural stigma not only informs tragic practices, it also manifests itself in the way medical professionals work with Black people and other members of non-dominant cultural groups. Research demonstrates that, as a result of factors including structural stigma, Black clients receive less information, empathy and attention from their doctors related to health and wellness when compared to their White counterparts (Russell et al., 2014). This structural stigma also provides context to understand why it took so long for the opioid epidemic to impact Black people when compared to White America's early adoption.

Opium was widely used after the American Civil War, and cocaine increased in popularity later in the 1800s. Opium and Cocaine epidemics plagued urban and rural centers across America toward the end of the 1800s, so much so that local governments began to prohibit opium use and distribution. After the Civil War, many soldiers had become addicted to the commonly used pain killer morphine. Morphine was highly depended upon due to the lack of alternatives for pain tolerance following gun wounds and amputations. Addiction to morphine among the soldiers was so common that it was referred to as the Soldiers Disease. The major treatment for opium addiction was morphine which was considered less addictive or even non-addictive according to some reports from the time. In the late 1990s, pharmaceutical companies ensured the public and the medical community that managing people's pain with opioids was now truly safe and that the likelihood of addiction was low, unlike the opioids of the prior century. As a result, health care providers began distributing opioids widely (Narconon).

In the late 1990s, it is estimated that upward of 100 million people were affected by some form of chronic pain. Between 1991 and 2011, US prescriptions for pain killers grew by over 300% (Hoffman, Trawalter, Axt, & Oliver, 2016). Research demonstrates that when compared to White consumers, Black consumers are less likely to be given pain medication and when administration does occur, doses and/or quantities are lower. In order to experiment on Black bodies, science convinced itself that Black people, in some cases, had a higher tolerance for pain and punishment than other humans and in other cases don't deserve proper treatment for their pain due to a propensity to misuse pain management medication. As a result, Black Americans experiencing chronic pain during this time were forced to endure their pain absent pharmacological intervention or to identify other non-government regulated chemicals to relieve the pain for which others were granted prescriptions (Hoffman et al., 2016).

Substance Abuse and Mental Health Services Administration reports that since 1999, opiate overdose deaths have increased 265% among men and 400% among women. In the last decade, US heroin use—an opioid—has risen exponentially (Centers for Disease Control [CDC]). Due to a history of structural stigma that ignored the pain of beleaguered Black bodies through violation and experimentation, heroin dependence has increased primarily among White Americans. Whites 18–44 represent the largest population of and the largest increase in US heroin addiction, although recent numbers demonstrate a rapid increase of opioid addiction among Black Americans. It is yet to be seen if the growing numbers of Black opiate addicts will be granted the same access to the empathic life-saving and generation preserving systems of support afforded to their earlier White counterparts (National Academies of Sciences, Engineering, and Medicine, 2017).

Perceived and tangible barriers related to one's ability to access services within or outside their community play a significant role in help seeking behavior, utilization of available services and efficacy of service rendered. Understanding the factors that influence how Black men perceive supportive and rehabilitation services for mental, somatic and behavioral health is important to understanding data on utilization and access. In order to appropriately address the risk factors associated with inequities in access for Black men, it is necessary to address each ecological system in which the risks exist. Individuals of African descent and from Black and minority ethnic (BME) communities across the world tend to have "poorer health outcomes (and) a shorter life expectancy" (Memon et al., 2016, pp. 1–2). According to this same study, these groups also experience more difficulty in accessing healthcare and mental health services when compared to the majority of the populations.

The Black Minority and Ethnic Community Partnership (BMECP) is a non-profit organization in the UK that works with the BME communities to create supportive infrastructures aimed at community cohesion.

In Southeast England, researchers partnered with their local BMECP center to hold focus groups on service access perceptions among Black Brits and other BME. The data collected from the focus groups would be used to influence the development and authorization of practices that were both effective and "culturally acceptable" for the non-White citizens of Britain. This study was commissioned by the UK's Department of Health's Delivering Race Equality in Mental Healthcare program. The results of this study identified two major themes associated with perceived barriers to mental health access for BME's in the UK. In addition to financial factors and wait times, the two interrelated major themes were broken down into sub-themes.

Table 6.1 was created using data from the UK's Department of Health's Delivering Race Equality in Mental Healthcare program.

Table 6.1 Self-report of perceived mental health access and utilization barriers for BME in the UK (Memon et al., 2016)

Major themes	
Personal and environmental factors	*Relationship between service user and healthcare provider*
Sub-themes	Sub-themes
Recognition of mental health problems: Inability to recognize symptoms of mental illness and/or unwillingness to accept a diagnosis of mental illness.	Responsiveness to needs: Participants describe a focus on medication to the exclusion of other complimentary approaches.
Social networks: Networks of families and friends can provide a safe space for discussing problems and worries creating a perceived adequate substitute for professional services.	Communication: Inability of doctors to listen to specific concerns and the use of a generalized approach to treatment with the same plan for each client.
Gender differences: Men were less likely to engage in services, felt excluded from services and ascribed a value to self-reliance as a mediator to mental wellness concerns.	Awareness of services: Participants indicated a lack of awareness regarding the availability of varied community wellness services available to them.
Cultural identity: Ethnic identity and associated stigma place an undue burden of historical context on an individual's ability to access services.	Cultural naivety, insensitivity and discrimination: Participants described their providers as unable to understand their experiences and uncomfortable discussing racism and discrimination.
	Manifestation power and authority: Clients report feeling like they were being "talked down to".

Morbid Epidemiology

Although lung cancer appears to be more deadly than other cancers, prostate cancer is the most common cancer occurring in men in the UK, the USA, France and Canada. Black men in the UK are two to three times more likely to develop it and twice as likely to die from it than their White male counterparts. Age-adjusted incidence rate for Black men in the UK is 647 per 100,000, compared to 213 for Whites and 213 for Asians (Canadian Cancer Society; Nderitu et al., 2016). In 2016, cancer epidemiologists looked at data sets for over 200,000 men to assess how socio-demographic, lifestyle and health-related characteristics contributed to their propensity to engage in prostate-specific antigen (PSA) testing in the UK. In this sample, the Black men were more likely to have had a PSA test when compared to their White male counterparts (Littlejohns, Travis, Key, & Allen, 2016). This is certainly a protective factor related to the prevention and early intervention models of wellness. PSA testing at the prescribed age and under the appropriate conditions is rarely contraindicated.

Although research on prostate cancer loosely implicates a myriad of socio-demographic, behavioral and nutritional factors, there are two very well-established risk factors: African ethnic descent and family history. It was determined that men who lived in socio-economically deprived areas were current smokers, had high BMI, have had heart disease or a stroke or had been diagnosed with diabetes were all less likely to have had a PSA test. The generalizability of this study is demonstrated by the disproportionate representation of Black men in each of those aforementioned areas. Black men in these four nations are more likely than White men to grow and develop in socio-economically disadvantaged communities and experience the associated risk factors. Black men are highly representative in samples of global smokers and persons living with diabetes. Black men are also more likely to experience strokes and suffer from heart disease than their White counterparts.

Unlike prostate cancer, other cancer types are attributable to modifiable risk factors like smoking/chewing tobacco, eating poorly, consuming alcohol heavily and leading a sedentary life style. For men in France, the UK, Canada and the USA, lung cancer sits atop this list and smoking is the biggest risk. In 2015, the rate of new cancer diagnoses for Black men in America was 501 for every 100,000 people; it was 469 and 352 for White and Hispanic Americans, respectively. Limited-duration prevalence is the number of people alive on a certain day who were diagnosed with a disease during a specified number of years. The estimated prevalence percentage for US Black men in their 60s was 6.12% compared to 4.92 for White men in the USA (Centers for Disease Control [CDC]).

Population-attributable fractions (PAF) are used in epidemiology research to quantify the proportion of incidents of a particular condition that are attributable to a specific set of risk factors. In a 2015 study, a PAF for tobacco smoking was established using lung cancer rates in France that were bifurcated between smokers and non-smokers. Researchers found that 41% (142,000) of all French cancer cases recorded were attributable to the identified modifiable factors, with smoking representing 20% of that total. The leading causes of new incidences of cancer among French men in 2015 were tobacco smoking (28.5%), alcohol (8.5%) and dietary factors (5.7%) (Soerjomataram et al., 2018). Recent research published in the International Journal of Cancer found that socio-economic environment as measured by the European Deprivation Index (EDI) played a significant role in age-standardized net survival (ASNS). Although the causes of cancer incident disparity related to social deprivation are not all understood, research has identified that the people who experience poverty and cancer are at a more advanced stage when diagnosed and have limited access to healthcare, fewer treatment choices, high prevalence of comorbid disorders and engage in more frequent lifestyle activities that hold carcinogenic risks (Tron, Dejardin, Launoy, & Beot, 2019).

Even though Black Americans' self-reported cancer diagnoses are lower than that of Whites, African Americans are dying from these diseases more frequently. This evidence demonstrates that cancer in Black men is far more deadly than in most other ethnic groups. In addition to other factors, researchers included the residential segregation of Blacks, the internalization by Blacks of overall society's negative characterization of them and the psychological stress resulting from experiences of interpersonal racism and discrimination as explanations for Black–White health inequities (Veenstra & Patterson, 2016).

The most common cardiovascular diseases include coronary artery disease (atherosclerosis), hypertension (high blood pressure), congestive heart failure, congenital heart disease, heart attack and stroke. They often involve narrowed or blocked blood vessels or conditions that affect the muscles in your heart or its valves. Black Canadians and Americans are less likely to report heart disease but more likely to report hypertension. This seeming paradox operationalizes itself in the USA through higher mortality rates attributed to cardiovascular disease for American Blacks than American Whites. Serious concern is warranted when one group hosts a lower number of diagnosed instances of a disorder or condition but experience a higher rate of death in that same category. This means that hypertension is disproportionately deadly in Black Americans and Canadians when compared to their White counterparts (Veenstra & Patterson, 2016).

Abnormal trabecular patterns in the myocardium of the heart's ventricles exist with cardiac disease and general aging. Researchers using data from cardiac magnetic resonance imaging confirmed an association between increased left ventricular endocardial complexity among Black patients. These complexities are a part of the endocardial remodeling process associated with heart failure. Atrial Fibrillation (AF) has become a significant public health concern due to its pervasiveness and mortality. Risk factors of AF including hypertension, stroke, heart failure, diabetes and stroke—all disproportionately represented among Black men—are responsible for 58% of AF burden in African Americans (only 44% in Whites) (Soerjomataram et al., 2018). In a study on a predictive risk model for incidences of AF, the researchers determined that Black men in both the USA and Europe demonstrated a significantly higher five-year predictive risk for the disorder (Alonso et al., 2013). Several studies demonstrated that Black men, although overall less likely to actually develop AF, are more likely to die when they do and have significantly worse outcomes with the associated conditions. "The absolute risk of developing stroke, heart failure, coronary artery disease, or all-cause mortality in AF patients was greater for Black individuals than White individuals" (Stamos & Darbar, 2016). These unexplained cardiovascular phenomena continue to be strongly correlated to socio-economic factors, neighborhood social environments and other associated adverse health events.

In 2014, the World Health Organization estimated that 422 million people across the world suffered from diabetes; this is a jump of almost 400% from the 108 million people estimated in 1980 (World Health Organization, 2016). Black citizens of Britain, the USA, France and Canada each experience higher rates of diabetes and death as a result of complications from diabetes than their White counterparts in each of these nations. Note that 8.3% of all people in the USA suffer from diabetes, among them are African Americans who are over-represented in hosting risk factors associated with diagnosis, frequency of diagnoses in population and morbidity from disease sequelae. Black people in America are 80% more likely to be diagnosed with diabetes by a physician, 4.2%

more likely to be diagnosed with diabetic nephropathy or end stage renal disease, 3.5 times more likely to experience a diabetes-related amputation and twice as likely to die from diabetes. Although African Americans suffering from diabetes often have lower aggregate rates of cardiovascular disease, their death rates associated with diabetes remain due to heart disease and strokes at a higher rate than their non-Hispanic White male counterparts (Spanakis & Golden, 2013; US Department of Health and Human Services). Researchers have explored the impact of chronic stressors like life-long race-based discrimination, internalized oppression and insulin resistance to explain some of these disparities in African American men and diabetes.

The prevalence of diabetes in France is the highest of all chronic conditions covered in full by the statutory health insurance (SHI) established in 2010. At 6%, the number of covered patients doubled in just one decade. In France, diabetes is the primary cause of adult blindness, amputation and dialysis along with a host of other medical conditions. The leading cause of death for individuals with diabetes in France is cardiovascular disease. One study of individuals receiving dialysis treatments for diabetes in France provided a diabetes prevalence map across the 22 administrative regions of the country. The researchers did not disaggregate the data based on ethnicity or cultural tradition resulting in challenges determining the prevalence among French people of African origin. Through extrapolations based on the geographic distribution and known demographics in those regions, this study was able to make some anecdotal conclusions regarding the ethnic ancestry of those communities most disproportionately impacted by diabetes throughout the country (Halimi et al., 1999).

Diseases that are linked to unhealthy behaviors are among the leading causes of male mortality and morbidity across the world. Cardiovascular disease, hypertension, obesity, diabetes and cancer are all linked to common behaviors like smoking, heavy alcohol consumption, corrupted sleep habits, unhealthy diet and sedentary lifestyles. *Unhealthy Behaviors, Men and Comorbidities* (Punjani et al., 2018) found statistically significant relationships between behaviors and conditions or diseases, even when no research-based causal relationship existed (i.e. alcohol and hypertension).

Table 6.2 summarizes the findings from the 2018 Unhealthy Behaviors, Men and Comorbidities study.

Table 6.2 Unhealthy behaviors and comorbidity in Canadian men (Punjani et al., 2018)

Disease/condition	Predictive behavior(s)	Selected explanation(s)
Cardiovascular disease	Smoking, exercise	Exercise has beneficial effects on low and high density lipoproteins (LDL and HDL), and triglyceride levels
Hypertension	Sleep, alcohol, exercise	Aerobic exercise supplies an array of favorable factors to blood pressure
Diabetes	Smoking	Smoking impacts insulin resistance and inflammation
Diabetes	Smoking, eating	Diet can be used as a preventative measure to reduce adiposity, decrease insulin resistance and decrease glycemic indexes
Depression	Smoking, sleep, eating	Altered protein diets can affect dopamine availability resulting from lowered amounts of amino acids to break down
Osteoarthritis	Smoking	Smoking may impact joint cartilage by increased oxidant stress, tissue hypoxia and inhibition of cell proliferation

Mental health concerns are among the biggest and most dangerously tabooed topics among Black people across the diaspora. A comedian once said that the only mental condition that has ever existed in the Black community was "a nervous breakdown". This speaks to the millions of people of African descent in the shadows suffering alone, managing the weight of the world in silent bent knee prayer. Some believe that if we ignore it for long enough or fail to name it, it will magically disappear. We know this is not true.

Canada's Black Health Alliance works to incorporate a culturally empathic lens through which mental wellness is seen. They integrate racism, discrimination and social injustices as severe risks to the disparities of Canada's Black population. The National Alliance on Mental Illness (NAMI) reports that Black Americans are 20% more likely to suffer from a serious mental health issue but half as likely to access mental health services when compared to White or Asian Americans. Arday (Arday, 2018) reports that Blacks experience significant disparity in mental healthcare pathways in the UK. This disparity manifests itself as fewer referrals to mental health services from their general practitioners and the increased likelihood of being "arrested by the police following a crisis, which inevitably results in poorer health outcomes and often coercive forms of care in locked wards" (Arday, 2018, p. 2). In the UK, "Black men are over-represented at the coercive end of the mental health system but under-represented in terms of seeking help voluntarily" (Arday, 2018, p. 3). A major underlying concern in global Black mental health is the lack of Black representation. Representation in research (both as investigator and participant), in the clinician's chair, on the clinics board of directors and among in-patient facility C-suite executives is significantly lacking. "The imbalance in representation indirectly perpetuates existing power imbalances and inequities" which result in reduced access to certain types of therapeutic interventions, over emphasis of pharmacological interventions and incorrect diagnoses (Arday, 2018). Each of these factors create a huge systemic gap in wellness opportunities for communities that experience a unique set of oppressive stressors that negatively impact somatic and behavioral health.

In 1964, Dr. Martin Luther King Jr. wrote:

> White Americans must be made to understand the basic motives underlying Negro demonstrations. Many pent-up resentments and latent frustrations are boiling inside the Negro, and he must release them. It is not a threat but a fact of history that if an oppressed people's pent up emotions are not nonviolently released they will be violently released. So let the Negro march. Let him make pilgrimages to city hall. Let him go on freedom rides. And above all, make an effort to understand why he must do this. For if his frustration and despair are allowed to continue piling up, millions of Negroes will seek solace and security in the Black-nationalist ideologies. And this, inevitably, would lead to a frightening racial nightmare. (Adler, 1968, p. 137)

Some refer to the summers of the mid-1960s as The Long Hot Summers. There were hundreds of riots and uprisings all across the country, and people were sick and tired of being mistreated and wanted their voices heard. Blacks across the country demanded equal access to jobs, education and housing. They demanded equal treatment from and protection by the police. They demanded the basic civil rights due to them. In July of 1967, America saw one of its worse riots ever. In the five days that it lasted, over 40 people died and thousands were injured and arrested. During the years of the 1960s, while Blacks were raising their voices in both civil and uncivil disobedience, the American Psychiatric Association was revising the DSM (1952) to the DSM II, publicized as a more scientific and objective document than its predecessor. In the DSM II (1968), the criteria and population most often diagnosed with "schizophrenic reaction" made a terse and abrupt transition.

"One of the most consistent research findings related to race and diagnosis is the disproportionately high rate of psychotic disorder diagnoses among consumers of color, specifically African Americans" (Schwartz & Blankenship, 2014, p. 134). Ionia State Hospital was opened in 1885 under its original name, the Michigan Asylum for Insane Criminals. Although all patients had not been convicted of crimes, many were felons from other prisons who had been sent there. Today, Black men in the USA and the UK are over-represented in the diagnosis of schizophrenia and other psychotic disorders. Black Americans are five times more likely to be diagnosed with schizophrenia compared to White Americans being admitted into psychiatric facilities. This remains true, even in the absence of any biogenetic data indicating an actual increase in population incidences. This hospital just west of Grand Rapids hold the records for what some believe was the genesis of this current diagnostic disproportionality.

Jonathan Metzl, author of *The Protest Psychosis: How Schizophrenia Became a Black Disease* (Metzl, 2010), reviewed the charts of over 800 patients who called the hospital home during its existence. The racial and gender diagnostic shifts were so striking that it became the central narrative for his text. He indicates that prior to the 1960s schizophrenia was primarily diagnosed in "nonviolent, White, petty criminals", including the hospital's considerable population of women from rural Michigan. Charts emphasized the negative impact on these women's ability to perform their "motherly duties". When the DSM II was released, the diagnostic frame for schizophrenia now included a "masculinized belligerence" characterized by a hostility and aggression consistent with existing delusions. Metzl noted that for many of the White women in the facility, their diagnoses of schizophrenic reaction were crossed out and largely replaced with depression and anxiety diagnoses. For the growing numbers of Black men being brought in from metro Detroit, their diagnosis was the new schizophrenia, paranoid subtype specifically (Metzl, 2010).

Mental wellness and illness are constructs largely defined by a set of expert's ability to agree on the meaning of ease or dis-ease. When members of the professional order are unable to come to agreement on who has a particular disorder or even a disorder at all, the public is placed in danger and opportunities for inequities grow. Concerns with interrater reliability exist with any multi-disciplinary and multi-phasic observations by people trained in different places at different times. Even when professionals are trained together by the same curriculum and instructors, drift from model fidelity is highly likely. One of the major benefits of the DSM V is the structuring of decision making processes to enhance agreement and improve consistency in the application of practices across areas of mental wellness. Citizens of African descent in each of the four nations in this study experience poorer outcomes related to key social and health indicators when compared to their counterparts of White European descent. In addition to the culturally and ethnically based prejudices they experience on a regularly basis, they are more likely to be diagnosed with psychotic disorders, are over-represented in in-patient psychiatric settings and are disproportionately misdiagnosed among other concerns (Metzl, 2010). In addition, these same groups have a lower mental health utilization rate than their White counterparts. Research demonstrates challenges in disaggregating whether or not these differences are related to a variance in the actual prevalence of mental health needs or if they are reflective of "institutional, cultural and/or socioeconomic exclusion factors" (Memon et al., 2016, p. 2).

Misdiagnosing remains a significant concern among Black boys and men. Whether in somatic medical care facilities, behavioral health care centers, penal industrial complexes or academic institutions, the dangers of misdiagnosed conditions can result in irreparable consequences. There are countless ways in which we see the folly of misdiagnoses play out across multiple disciplines at the intersection of Black maleness. In one instance, there is the practitioner's minimization of symptomology that renders children without adequate interventions for disorders and conditions whose morbidity and prognosis are dependent upon early detection and intervention. In other cases, the practitioner hypothesizes scenarios and explains symptomology through a stereotypical lens that paints the boy and his family into a self-fulfilling trajectory guided or misguided by a system mechanized to marginalize.

There are many correlations to mental wellness and socio-cultural disparities. Evidence from juvenile arrests shows that Black youth are three times more likely to be arrested than White youth. Some believe that the discrepancies in arrest rates are a reflection of Black youth exposure to environmental and societal inequities that result in the exhibition of amplified adverse risks associated with greater probability for arrest (Fite, Wyn, & Pardini, 2009). Research has identified a set of clinically specific risk factors across several domains that aggregate to support juvenile arrests. Many of these risk factors include either a disproportionate number of Black boys or a growth rate for Black boys that is exponentially faster than for other groups. Attention-deficit/hyperactivity problems, oppositional defiant problems, affective problems and interpersonal callousness have been associated with juvenile arrests across ethnicities.

Attention Deficit Hyperactivity Disorder (ADHD) is defined by the DSM V as a persistent pattern of inattention and/or hyperactivity-impulsivity that interferes with functioning or development as characterized by six or more "inattention" symptoms and/or six or more "hyperactivity/impulsivity" symptoms. The DSM V provides a prevalence rate in most cultures of about 5% in children and 2.5% of adults. Over a ten-year period (2001 to 2010), Kaiser Permanente Southern California conducted a study where they examined the electronic medical records of 850,000 ethnically diverse children ages five to eleven years. Overall, White children are diagnosed with ADHD more often than children of most other race, but the growth across this period was certainly different. "Black children showed the greatest increase in ADHD incidence, from 2.6 percent of all Black children 5 to 11 years of age in 2001 to 4.1% in 2010, a 70 percent increase." The study also found that boys were three times more likely to be diagnosed than girls and that families who earned more than $30,000 per year were 20% more likely to be diagnosed than those who make below $30,000 (Kaiser Permanente, 2013).

Boys in general, Black boys specifically, learn differently than what traditional schools offer. The model that requires students to sit still in their seats and work or read has been determined ineffective for working with young boys who might need to explore and may not want to sit in their seats while they read their book. Dr. Donna Ford, professor of human development at Vanderbilt, expressed her fears regarding the increasing trend of Black diagnoses and the potentiality of congruent rates of misdiagnosis. In a 2018 New York op-ed, she wrote "… boys tend to be more active than girls, and African Americans are known for being movement oriented, tactile and kinesthetic. This is considered normal and healthy in the African American community but not necessarily so in schools" (Ford, 2016).

The DSM V defines Oppositional Defiant Disorder (ODD) as "a pattern of angry/irritable mood, argumentative/defiant behavior, or vindictiveness lasting at least six months as evidenced by at least four symptoms" observed in a child of any age. Intermittent Explosive Disorder (IED) is diagnosed in children over six when observed demonstrating recurrent "behavioral outbursts representing a failure to control aggressive impulses" as confirmed by the types of aggression and the frequency of outbursts over a given time period. Conduct Disorder (CD) is a "repetitive and persistent pattern of behavior in which the basic rights of others or major age appropriate societal norms or rules have been violated". To meet criteria for the disorder, the individual must have violated at least 3 of the 15 identified societal rules that are stratified across 4 categories: Aggression to People and Animals, Destruction of Property, Deceitfulness or Theft and Serious Violations of the Rules.

Evidence of environmental impacts continues to show up in the literature and speaks to disparities in our people serving systems. The research concluded that "increased exposure to childhood risk factors across multiple domains accounted for racial differences" in initial and later arrests of the youth who participated in the study (Fite et al., 2009). These boys who were disproportionately represented in the juvenile adjudication systems were also disproportionately represented in the groups of children who experienced diagnoses of ADHD, ODD, IED and symptoms associated with apathy or callousness. The authors of these and other research studies insist that Black disproportionality is caused by the symptoms that Black youth display from engagement in the dangerous ecologies in which they are placed. The studies, however, seem to rest on a level of confidence in the diagnoses provided and their etiologies that many researchers are not comfortable with.

Many incarcerated men will identify a juvenile arrest as their initial foray into the criminal justice system. For many, their juvenile and adult arrest records are associated with one or more mental health conditions including ADHD, ODD, IED, CD and Antisocial Personality Disorder. Although the DSM V provides a clear and concise rubric from which symptomology can be selected to identify a proper clinical diagnosis, the clinical disproportionality remains prevalent. It is possible that the over-representation of Black boys in the juvenile justice system is not in fact due to a credible diagnosis based upon the youth's actual symptomology as some research asserts. In *Racial and Ethnic Disparities in ADHD Diagnosis from Kindergarten to Eighth Grade* (Morgan, Staff, Hillemeier, Farkas, & Maczuga, 2013), researchers found that Black and other minority children were less likely than White children to be diagnosed with ADHD and were less likely to engage in a pharmacological treatment for the disorder when it was diagnosed. The researchers conclude that this phenomenon exists due to a lack of culturally sensitive monitoring in the screening and diagnosing of Black boys. An alternative perspective demonstrates that these Black boys are still being diagnosed, just not in the Neurodevelopmental Disorder cluster where ADHD and specific learning disorders live (Morgan et al., 2013).

The cluster of disorders that make up Disruptive, Impulse-Control and Conduct Disorders in the DSM V are the most highly represented mental health conditions in prisons and other forensic settings. There are also certainly substance abuse concerns, mood disorders and an array of serious psychiatric concerns that contribute to experiences with incarceration. Many of them have co-morbidity with this cluster of diagnoses that often represent a road map to a life of incarceration. The over diagnoses of Black youth with disruptive disorders represent a rung on the school to prison pipeline.

An early diagnosis of ODD, IED or CD can have a devastating effect on a youth's entire life's trajectory. Self-Fulfilling Prophecy is often immediately enlisted in situations where these diagnoses exist. This construct indicates that the performance of the youth will be influenced at best and dictated at worst, by the expectations placed upon him. Adolescents are in increased danger of meeting low expectations when behaviors of others appear to confirm their alleged cognitive deficit, impulse dyscontrol or disruptive behavior patterns. Many of these youth were criminalized before they were born and have been treated accordingly. It is then systematized at their first offense—which for many is no longer a crime in contemporary times—resulting in an assembly line existence where the widgets are special education, medication, institutionalization and incarceration. In these scenarios, clinicians must help the adolescent using cognitive restructuring and eliminating cognitive distortions created by the inappropriately restrictive environment. This can prove to be a difficult task as the adolescent may have, through the process of self-fulfilling prophecy, developed a sense of himself built atop the foundation of a non-credible diagnosis grounded in stereotypes and culturally unempathic practices.

The experiences of Black families with Autistism Spectrum Disorder (ASD) diagnoses provide yet another demonstration of the misguided diagnoses that have long-lasting consequences on the lives of Black families and communities. Increasing evidence is demonstrating the effectiveness of clinical practices and tools that allow for the detection and identification of Autism in very young children, yet diagnosis is too often delayed until the children are school aged. In *Disparities in Diagnoses Received Prior to a Diagnosis of Autism Spectrum Disorder* (Mandell, Ittenbach, Levy, & Pinto-Martin, 2006), researchers looked at the different diagnoses that children were given prior to the final determination that they met criteria for Autism Spectrum Disorder (ASD). Assessing this data is critical given that prognoses for the future functionality and independence of children with pervasive developmental disorders are largely predicated upon early intervention, which requires an early and accurate diagnosis. In addition to delays in treatment as a result of misdiagnoses, the actual incorrect diagnosis selected by the practitioner(s) also makes a noteworthy statement. In this sample, Black children were 2.6 times less likely than White children to be diagnosed with Autism on their first visit to a specialist. Although ADHD was the most common diagnosis given instead of the actual ASD diagnosis, Black children were 5.1 times more likely to be misdiagnosed with adjustment disorder and 2.4 times more likely to be diagnosed with conduct disorder than ADHD when compared to their White counterparts. Past research demonstrated that, on average, Black children begin receiving care from specialists later than other children, received the ASD diagnosis 1.4 years later than White children and participated in eight more months of services under the care of a mental health professional before being diagnosed (Mandell et al., 2006).

Research indicates that 2500 African Americans died by suicide between 2010 and 2017 (Hollingsworth, Patton, Allen, & Johnson, 2018). Racism and discrimination have long been described as significant risk factors for suicide and depression, but recent research has increased focus on racial micro-aggressions as another likely contributor. Racial microaggressions are "verbal, behavioral, and environmental racist slights or insults directed to a person who is an ethnic minority group member" (Hollingsworth et al., 2018, p. 105). They occur in daily exchanges and, as research demonstrates, are experienced by people of African descent far more frequently than any other ethnic minority. These experiences are often so prevalent and frequent that they go undetected or are excused by the conscious mind, but not the subconscious. Racial microaggressions might be categorized into six dimensions: invisibility, criminality, low achieving/undesirable culture, sexualization, foreigner/not belonging and environmental invalidations.

Although data suggests that men and Blacks experience lower overall rates of depressive symptomology, research demonstrates that young Black men experience depressive symptoms at rates similar to or higher than White men and women (Kogan, Cho, Oshri, & Mackillop, 2017). Blacks are also more likely than Whites to rate their conditions as more severe, disabling and persistent in nature when compared to their White counterparts. As a consequence, mental health disorders and conditions among Black men are often a part of a dangerously synergistic dyad of chronicity and neglect. The fact that Black suicide rates have historically been low when compared to other groups is a dangerous statistic when left uncontextualized. From 1981 to 1994, Black suicide in America grew by a ghastly 83% (Grant Jr., 2013). In 2002, African American males died by suicide at a rate of 9.1 per 100,000 compared to 19.9 per 100,000 for European American males. Suicide is the third leading cause of death for Black males between the ages of 10 and 24 in America, and homicide is first for most of this group. These factors are replaced by cancer, heart disease and stroke for Black American men over the age of 55 (CDC).

WEAPONIZED NARCOTICS

Although America's first federal stance on substance abuse targeted doctors and pharmacists, it is not hard to see the streams of stigma and bias that flow through the history of substance abuse, drug addiction policy and rehabilitative practices. The US Harrison Narcotics Act of 1914 created restrictions and policies related to the production and sale of marijuana, cocaine, heroin and morphine. Thousands of doctors were imprisoned and fined into the 1930s as a result of the act and associated court actions. In 1930, the Federal Bureau of Narcotics was created which would facilitate a systemic increase in the criminalization of drugs, the individuals that use them and the families they come from. Around this same time, the American Psychiatric Association (APA) created its definition of substance use and abuse that incorporated aspects of the law. In 1952, the first edition of APA's Diagnostic and Statistical Manual of Mental Disorders (DSM) categorized substance abuse with sociopathic personality disturbances.

Legislation in the late 1950s may have stifled the growth of abuse and abusers, but the 1960s would birth a new movement. Marijuana, LSD and heroin were some of the most popular drugs of the 1960s. The Narcotics Addict Rehabilitation Act of 1966 identified drug abuse as a mental illness, although they continued to criminalize use, abuse and the abusers. This marked one of the first efforts to place dollars toward the treatment of addiction. Although the medical model of addiction for alcoholism existed, it was now for the first time being applied to narcotics.

Cannabis had been grown and used in the USA since the 1850s but wasn't used broadly as a recreational drug until after 1910. Even after its inception and acceptance as a recreational substance, it was primarily used for medicinal purposes while its strong fibers had long been valued in the creation of rope and other materials. The racial vilification of cannabis took a bimodal approach stratified both by ethnicity and geography. The anti-immigrant stance of the early twentieth century—strikingly similar to that of the early twenty-first century—created the Mexican cannabis caricature: a super-human, blood thirsty, Mexican criminal. America even strategically transitioned the colloquial nomenclature from cannabis to the Mexican "marihuana", a word only used consistently in American media after the early 1900s. Marijuana in the USA would later be linked to East coast and Southern Blacks, particularly through the jazz association. It was reported that marijuana could be purchased at "tea pads" across the country and was seen as an alternative to alcohol during prohibition in the 1920s. Marijuana use was strategically associated with jazz, Blacks, Mexicans, poverty and violence resulting in the Marijuana Tax Act of 1937 which criminalized the drug.

The early 1970s saw the introduction of both the temperance models and the disease models of addiction. These views laid the groundwork for the government funding of controversial and experimental programs aimed at rehabilitation and adjudication. In 1973, The Drug Enforcement Agency (DEA) was created and worked to impact Mexican marijuana production. For many, these regulations mark the systemic efforts to utilize substance possession and abuse as another entry portal to the revolving system of incarceration. Today, publically traded cannabis companies like Aurora and Canopy Growth are poised to foster and sustain an industry estimated to function at the multi-billion-dollar level. One that just less than a decade before was locking Black and Latinx adolescents up for grams of weed (Frontline, PBS).

Conditions like anxiety and depression have been described as both a cause and consequence of substance use and abuse. The self-medication hypothesis suggests that substance use serves as a mediator of and modulator for pre-existing emotions related to anxiety, depression and an array of other mental wellness concerns. Other studies identify other motives for the commencement and escalation of substance use and abuse non-inclusive of paradigms from the self-medication model. These reasons include but are not limited to social positioning, self-indulgent pleasure seeking and influences from peers (Kogan et al., 2017). Substance use and substance abuse disorders hold both correlational and causal relationships to a vast array of outcomes for all people. Health and wellness outcomes like early death, chronic pain, communicable diseases, accidents, high-risk sexual behaviors and mental health disorders along with socio-cultural outcomes related to vocational functioning, community death and incarceration taxes, crime, healthcare costs/debt and homelessness are all implicated among substance abuse concerns (Kogan et al., 2017; Vasilenko, Evans-Polce, & Lanza, 2018). Cross-sectional data demonstrate that the adverse outcomes of substance use and abuse are heightened for Black men, especially those from under-resourced communities where many members are also experiencing poverty in both rural and urban communities (Kogan et al., 2017; Vasilenko et al., 2018).

In the USA, 14% of people meet the minimum criteria for Alcohol Use Disorder (AUD), 13% for Tobacco Use Disorder (TUD), 4% for cannabis use disorder and 1% for Opioid Use Disorder. Blacks in the USA often demonstrate lower rates of AUDs, TUDs and OUDs when compared to their White counterparts. Although men do generally report a higher rate of substance use when compared to women, rates within ethnicity and among age groups demonstrate several noteworthy differences (Vasilenko et al., 2018).

For instance, Black adolescents have lower rates of substance use when compared to White adolescents, but this does not hold true into early adulthood, a time where Black emerging adults endorse higher usage of substances than do their White counterparts, particularly with respect to marijuana and alcohol (Kogan et al., 2017; Vasilenko et al., 2018). This time coincides with the transitions in life where the experiences with racism and discrimination have consequences that may hold more weight. Although Black boys and teens experience racism and discrimination, early adulthood is the time where oppression, for the first time, impacts their personal job opportunities, housing, socio-economic status and life's general course. This shift in existentially weighted responsibilities might hold some culpability in the change of endorsement for substance use.

The World Health Organization (2016) mentions alcohol abuse as one of the leading causes of morbidity and death across the globe. In 2004, almost 4% of worldwide deaths were attributed to alcohol. During this same year, "4.6% of the global burden of disease and injury, occurring mainly in individuals 15–30 years of age, was attributable to alcohol" (World Health Organization, 2016, p. 40). The majority of these alcohol-related ailments resulting in death were cancer, cardiovascular disease and cirrhosis. The vast majority of the alcohol-related deaths were of men.

Cirrhosis is the final stage of most all liver diseases, those associated with alcohol abuse and those not associated. Cirrhosis occurs as the functional tissues of the liver are damaged due to over use and are subsequently replaced by non-functional scar tissue. It is important to note the challenge in quantifying this correlation accurately given that the alcohol-attributable risks are rarely linear or operational in isolation. Some autopsy studies show that mortality data may include fewer than half of the cirrhosis deaths, while in another estimate, the percentage of cirrhotic deaths missed was above 60% (Stinson, Grant, & Dufour, 2001). In 1997, liver cirrhosis was the tenth leading cause of death in the USA. Although there has been an observable drop in deaths due to cirrhosis, it remains a critical area of disproportionality where Black men continue to die more frequently than any group, other than Hispanic men (Caetano, 2003).

Heavy drinking is often described in the research as five or more drinks during a single drinking event or occasion. When this occurs more than five times within a 30-day period, researchers often begin to look for and/ or identify specific alcohol-related problems. Alcohol-related problems refer to the varied troubles that often accompany individuals who drink heavily on a regular basis. Some of these problems are social concerns like divorce and job loss, others are legal like driving under the influence (DUI) of alcohol (or other drugs), criminal charges and incarceration, while others are physiological ramifications of alcohol dependence like body tremors and organ systems impairment. US studies indicate that Black American men have consistently maintained a general threshold of heavy drinking, a statistic that has declined among White American men over the past two decades (Caetano, 2003; Stinson et al., 2001). Intimate partner violence is one of the alcohol-related problems discussed throughout the literature on substance abuse. One report showed that, among Blacks, both male to female and female to male intimate partner violence was significantly higher than that of White and Hispanic Americans.

Black men are disproportionately represented in global systems of incarceration, among many other things, removing them from the statistical samples of research on outcomes in the general population of Black men. One possible result of this sampling concern could be related to the underestimation of Black men using prescription drugs for non-medical use and a subsequent lack of services dedicated to prevention, early intervention and treatment of prescription drug abuse among Black men. One study on the pre-incarceration rates of non-medical prescription drugs use

(NMPDU) among Black men found that the rates are likely much higher than the research demonstrates. Researchers also found that another limitation to current data was the urban nomenclature of many prescription drugs when compared to the names and labels used in the research studies. Codeine cough syrup might be referred to as "lean" or "syrup (or sizzurp)", while Amphetamines might be "Speed, Addies or Truck Drivers", and opiates might be "Percs, Oxy or Norco". In this study, almost 60% of the men reported taking prescription drugs that had not been prescribed to them or their proxy; this rate was highest among men between 30 and 39 years old. By far, cough syrup with codeine was the most frequently misused specific drug with Xanax and Lortab following. The most commonly used class of drugs were sedatives, hypnotics and tranquilizers followed in second by opioids and then amphetamines (Wheeler, Stevens-Watkins, Knighton, Mahaffey, & Lewis, 2018).

Conclusion

In 1951, Langston Hughes wrote about a dream deferred in the short poem entitled Harlem. In this poem, Hughes asks us, "What happens to a dream deferred?" He posits several potential outcomes: It might "dry up like a raisin in the sun" or "fester like a sore". In the final line of this short poem, after presenting several other options of a dream's fate, he asks a question that feels more like a prophetic statement. In his closing line he asks, "or does it explode?"

As I watch the events of today's world, I see the great grandchildren of Walter Lee, the lead character in Lorraine Hansberry's award-winning play "A Raisin in the Sun". Walter Lee watched dream after dream deferred living on the Southside of Chicago, as did Black men in New York, Los Angeles and Milwaukee during this same time in the 1960s. These men who watched their fathers recover (or not) from Jim Crow's lashings now have their own children watching the deferred dreams of their father's sag like heavy loads … right before they explode.

Proponents of Black exceptionalism reading this are likely thinking of all the families they know that migrated north and thrived. They left the Jim Crow South, bought their Cadillac, sent their children to an HBCU, watched their grandchildren grow up in Jack and Jill and head off to the Ivy League. These families are not unicorns, they are very present but in no way indicative of an environment void of insurmountable toxins, abuses and deliberately placed obstacles like under-resourced schools, crack cocaine, disparate distribution of justice and a privatized system of incarceration. Research clearly demonstrates a propensity for adversity to result in resiliency for a segment of those who experience it. But what about the others, those for whom deferred dreams are currently exploding right in front of us?

As these families experience compounding complex trauma and a true lack of hope, the rhetoric must stop and authentic change work must begin. This can only happen when we stop blaming the oppressed for the consequences of their oppression which is different from accountability. The prison industrial complex has turned into a modern slave quarter, and those who promote interventions grounded in a punitive lens are missing the mark. As we pour money into prisons and jails, we continue to expand the loss of fathers, grandfathers, uncles and nephews as contributing members to child and community development. If we don't reallocate dollars toward programs that fill the soul holes that adolescent boys and girls seek to fill through gang-membership, substance abuse, violence and criminality, we will continue to exacerbate the raging fire debilitating our communities across the globe.

References

Abell, J., Stadler, T., Ferrie, J., Shelby, M., Kirschbaum, C., Kivmaki, M., et al. (2016). Assessing Cortisol from Hair Samples in a Large Observational Cohort: The Whitehall II Study. *Psychoneuroendocrinology, 73*, 148–156.

Adler, B. (1968). *He Wisdom of Martin Luther King; In His Own Words*. New York: Lancer Books.

Alonso, A., Krijthe, B., Aspelund, T., Stepas, K., Pencina, M., Moser, et al. (2013). Simple Risk Model Predicts Incidence of Atrial Fibrillation in a Racially and Geographically Diverse Population: The CHARGE-AF Consortium. *Journal of the American Heart Association, 2*(2), e000102.

American Council on Education. (2012). *By the Numbers. More Black Men in Prison Than in College? Think Again*. Retrieved from https://www.acenet.edu/the-presidency/columns-and-features/Pages/By-the-Numbers-More-Black-Men-in-Prison-Than-in-College-Think-Again-.aspx

American Psychological Association. *Understanding Chronic Stress*. Retrieved from https://www.apa.org/helpcenter/understanding-chronic-stress

Arday, J. (2018). Understanding Mental Health: What Are the Issues for Black and Ethnic Minority Students at University? *Social Sciences, 7*, 196.

Bulhan, H. (2015). Stages of Colonialism in Africa: From Occupation of Land to Occupation of Being. *Journal of Social and Political Psychology, 3*(1), 239–256.

Caetano, R. (2003). Alcohol-Related Health Disparities and Treatment—Related Epidemiological Findings Among Whites, Blacks, and Hispanics in the United States. *Alcoholism: Clinical and Experiential Research, 27*(8), 1337–1339.

Canadian Cancer Society. *Cancer Statistics at a Glance*. Retrieved from http://www.cancer.ca/en/cancer-information/cancer-101/cancer-statistics-at-a-glance/?region=ab

Centers for Disease Control (CDC). (n.d.) *Health Equity Leading Causes of Death (LCOD) by Age Group*. Retrieved from https://www.cdc.gov/healthequity/lcod/men/2014/Black/index.htm

Centers for Disease Control (CDC). *Prescription Painkiller Overdoses*. Retrieved form https://www.cdc.gov/vitalsigns/prescriptionpainkilleroverdoses/index.html

Centers for Disease Control (CDC). *United States Cancer Statistics: Data Visualizations*. Retrieved form https://gis.cdc.gov/cancer/USCS/DataViz.html

Croizet, J.-C., Depres, G., & Gauzins, M.-E. (2004). Stereotype Threat Undermines Intellectual Performance by Triggering an Disruptive Mental Load. *Personality and Social Psychology Bulletin, 30*(6), 721–731.

Crosby, F., & Van de Veer, C. (Eds.). (2000). *Sex, Race, and Merit: Debating Affirmative Action in Education and Employment*. Ann Arbor, MI: The University of Michigan Press.

Desmond-Harris, J. (2015). *The Myth That There Are More Black Men in Prison Than in College, Debunked in One Chart*. Vox. Retrieved from https://www.vox.com/2015/2/12/8020959/Black-men-prison-college

Fite, P., Wyn, P., & Pardini, D. (2009). Explaining Discrepancies in Arrest Rates Between Black and White Male Juveniles. *Journal of Consulting and Clinical Psychology, 77*(5), 916–927.

Ford, D. (2016). Don't Rush to Saddle Children with the ADHD Label. *New York Times*. Retrieved from https://www.nytimes.com/roomfordebate/2016/02/01/is-the-adhd-diagnosis-helping-or-hurting-kids/dont-rush-to-saddle-children-with-the-adhd-label

Frontlines (PBS). *A Social History of America's Most Popular Drugs*. Retrieved from https://www.pbs.org/wgbh/pages/frontline/shows/drugs/buyers/socialhistory.html

Grand, J. (2016). Brain Drain? An Examination of Stereotype Threat Effects During Training on Knowledge Acquisition and Organizational Effectiveness. *Journal of Applied Psychology, 102*(2), 115–150.

Grant, Jr., D. E. (2013). Black Suicide When Prayer Isn't Enough. *Ebony Magazine*. Retrieved from https://www.ebony.com/health/Black-suicide-when-prayer-is-not-enough-405/

Halimi, S., Zmirou, D., Benhamou, P. Y., Balducci, F., Zaoui, P., Magihlaoua, M., et al. (1999). Huge Progression of Diabetes Prevalence and Incidence Among Dialysed Patients in Mainland France and Overseas French Territories. A Second National Survey Six Years Apart. (Uremidiab 2 Study). *Diabetes & Metabolism, 25*, 507–512.

Henley, P., Jahedmotlagh, Z., Thomas, S., Darnell, R., Jacobs, D., Johnson, J., et al. (2013). Hair Cortisol as a Biomarker of Stress Among a First Nation in Canada. *Therapeutic Drug Monitoring, 35*(5), 595–599.

Hockenbury, D., & Hockenbury, S. (2004). *Psychology.* New York: Worth Publishers.

Hoffman, K., Trawalter, S., Axt, J., & Oliver, M. N. (2016). Racial Bias in Pain Assessment and Treatment Recommendations, and False Beliefs About Biological Differences Between Blacks and Whites. *PNAS, 113*(16), 4296–4301.

Hollingsworth, L. D., Patton, D., Allen, P., & Johnson, K. (2018). Racial Microaggressions in Social Work Education: Black Students' Encounters in a Predominantly White Institution. *Journal of Ethnic & Cultural Diversity in Social Work, 1*, 95–105.

Honora, D. (2003). Urban African American Adolescents and School Identification. *Urban Education, 38*, 58–77.

Justice Policy Institute. (2002). *Cellblocks or Classroom: The Funding of Higher Education and Corrections and Its Impact on African American Men.* Retrieved from http://www.justicepolicy.org/uploads/justicepolicy/documents/02-09_rep_cellblocksclassrooms_bb-ac.pdf

Kaiser Permanente. (2013). *Kaiser Permanente Study Finds Childhood Diagnosis of ADHD Increased Dramatically Over Nine-Year Period.* Retrieved from https://www.prnewswire.com/news-releases/kaiser-permanente-study-finds-childhood-diagnosis-of-adhd-increased-dramatically-over-nine-year-period-187780921.html

Kenyon, P. (1994). Depression and Learned Helplessness. In *Study and Learning Material On-Line (SALMON).* Devon: University of Pennsylvania.

Kogan, S. M., Cho, J., Oshri, A., & Mackillop, J. (2017). The Influence of Substance Abuse on Depressive Symptoms Among Young Adult Black Men: The Sensitizing Effect of Early Adversity. *The American Journal of Addiction, 26*, 400–406.

Larry, P. v Riles. NO C-71-2270 RFP. 495 F. Supp. 926. United States District Court, N. D. California.

Littlejohns, T., Travis, R., Key, T., & Allen, N. (2016). Lifestyle Factors and Prostate-Specific Antigen (PSA) Testing in UK Biobank: Implications for Epidemiological Research. *International Journal of Cancer Epidemiology, Detection, and Prevention, 45*, 40–46.

Livingstone Smith, D. (2011). *Less Than Human: Why We Demean, Enslave, and Exterminate Others.* New York: St. Martin's Press.

Mandell, D. S., Ittenbach, R. F., Levy, S. E., & Pinto-Martin, J. A. (2006). Disparities in Diagnoses Received Prior to a Diagnosis of Autism Spectrum Disorder. *Journal of Autism and Developmental Disorders, 37*(9), 1795–1802.

Mantovani, N., Pizzolati, M., & Edge, D. (2017). Exploring the Relationship Between Stigma and Help-Seeking for Mental Illness in African-Descended Faith Communities in the UK. *Health Expectations, 20*(3), 373–384.

Memon, A., Taylor, K., Mohebati, L., Sundin, J., Cooper, M., Scanion, T., et al. (2016). Perceived Barriers to Accessing Mental Health Service Among Black and Minority Ethnic (BME) Communities: A Qualitative Study in Southeast England. *BJM Open, 6*(11), e012337.

Merl, J. (1991). Court Ban on IQ Tests for Blacks Sparks Parents' Suit. *LA Times.* Retrieved from http://articles.latimes.com/1991-08-05/news/mn-139_1_iq-test

Metzl, J. (2010). *The Protest Psychosis: How Schizophrenia Became a Black Disease.* Boston: Beacon Press.

Mills, A. J., Durepos, G., & Wiebe, E. (2010). *Encyclopedia of Case Study Research* (Vol. 1-0). Thousand Oaks, CA: SAGE.

Morgan, P., Staff, J., Hillemeier, M., Farkas, G., & Maczuga, S. (2013). Racial and Ethnic Disparities in ADHD Diagnosis from Kindergarten to Eighth Grade. *Pediatrics, 132*(1), 85.

Narconon. *Heroin History 1900's.* Retrieved from https://www.narconon.org/drug-information/heroin-history-1900s.html

National Academies of Sciences, Engineering, and Medicine. (2017). *Pain Management and the Opioid Epidemic: Balancing Societal and Individual Benefits and Risks of Prescription Opioid Use.* Washington, DC: National Academies Press.

National Alliance on Mental Illness. *African American Mental Health.* Retrieved from https://www.nami.org/Find-Support/Diverse-Communities/African-Americans

Nderitu, P., Van Hemelrijck, M., Ashworth, M., Mathur, R., Hull, S., Dudek, A., et al. (2016). Prostate-Specific Antigen Testing in Inner London General Practices: Are Those at Higher Risk Most Likely to Get Tested? *BMJ Open, 6*(7), e011356.

Punjani, N., Flannigan, R., Oliffe, J. L., McCreary, D. R., Black, N., & Larry Goldenberg, S. (2018). Unhealthy Behaviors Among Canadian Men Are Predictors of Comorbidities: Implications for Clinical Practice. *American Journal of Men's Health, 12*(6), 2183–2193.

Quijano, A., & Ennis, M. (2000). *Coloniality of Power, Eurocentrism and Latin America in Nepantla: Views from South 1(3)* (pp. 533–580). London: Duke University Press.

Rosenthal, R., & Jacobson, L. (1966). Teachers' Expectations: Determinates of Pupils' IQ Gains. *Psychological Reports, 19*, 115–118.

Russell, E., Koren, G., Rieder, M., & Van Uum, S. H. (2014). The Detection of Cortisol in Human Sweat: Implications for Measurement of Cortisol in Hair. *Therapeutic Drug Monitoring, 36*(1), 30–34.

Scharff, D., Matthews, K., Jackson, P., Hoffsuemmer, J., Emeobong, M., & Edwards, D. (2010). More Than Tuskegee: Understanding mistrust about research participation. *Journal of Health Care for the Poor and Underserved, 21*(3), 879–897. Johns Hopkins University Press.

Schwartz, R., & Blankenship, D. (2014). Racial Disparities in Psychotic Disorder Diagnosis: A Review of Empirical Literature. *World Journal of Psychiatry, 4*(4), 133–140.

Shields, K. (1997). *The Conflicts of Learned Helplessness in Motivation.* San Jose State University. Retrieved from http://ematusov.soe.udel.edu/final.paper.pub/_pwfsfp/00000062.htm

Soerjomataram, I., Sheild, K., Marant-Micallef, C., Vignat, J., Hill, C., Rogel, A., et al. (2018). Cancers Related to Lifestyle and Environmental Factors in France in 2015. *European Journal of Cancer, 105*, 103–113.

Spanakis, E. K., & Golden, S. H. (2013). Race/Ethnic Difference in Diabetes and Diabetic Complications. *Current Diabetes Reports, 13*(6), 814–823.

Stamos, T., & Darbar, D. (2016). The "Double" Paradox of Atrial Fibrillation in Black Individuals. *Journal of American Medicine Cardiology, 1*(4), 377–379.

Steele, C. M. (1997). A Threat in the Air: How Stereotypes Shape Intellectual Identity and Performance. *American Psychologist, 52*(6), 613–629.

Stinson, F. S., Grant, B. F., & Dufour, M. C. (2001). The Critical Dimension of Ethnicity in Liver Cirrhosis Mortality Statistics. *Alcoholics Clinical Experimental Research, 25*(8), 1181–1187.

The Anti-Slavery Monthly. (1828). On the Demoralizing Influence of Slavery. *Reporter, Jun.1825–Dec.1831, 2*(32), 176.

Thomas, M. (1986). The Use of Expectancy Theory and the Theory of Learned Helplessness in Building Strengths of Ethnic Minorities: The Black Experience in the United States. *International Journal for the Achievement of Counseling, 9*(4), 371–379.

Toldson, I. (2013). More Black Men in Jail Than in College? Wrong. *The Root.* Retrieved from https://www.theroot.com/more-Black-men-in-jail-than-in-college-wrong-1790895415

Tron, L., Dejardin, O., Launoy, G., & Beot, A. (2019). Socioeconomic Environment and Disparities in Cancer Survival for 19 Solid Tumor Sites: An Analysis of the French Network of Cancer Registries (FRANCIM) Data. *International Journal of Cancer, 144*(6), 1262–1274.

U.S. Department of Health & Human Services. *Diabetes and African Americans.* Retrieved from https://minorityhealth.hhs.gov/omh/browse.aspx?lvl=4&lvlid=18

Vasilenko, S., Evans-Polce, R., & Lanza, S. (2018). Age Trends in Rates of Substance Use Disorders Across Ages 18–90: Differences by Gender and Race/Ethnicity. *Journal of Drug and Alcohol Dependence, 180*(2017), 260–264.

Veenstra, G., & Patterson, C. (2016). Black-White Health Inequalities in Canada. *Journal of Immigrant Minority Health, 18*, 51–57.

Wheeler, P., Stevens-Watkins, D., Knighton, J. S., Mahaffey, C., & Lewis, D. (2018). Pre-incarceration Rates of Nonmedical Use of Prescription Drugs

Among Black Men from Urban Communities. *Journal of Urban Health,* *95*(4), 444–453.

World Health Organization. (2016). *Global Report on Diabetes.* WHO. Retrieved from https://apps.who.int/iris/bitstream/handle/10665/204871/ 9789241565257_eng.pdf;jsessionid=873C5E782CEE5ECE543CD8F76A5 1B2F7?sequence=1

Wyatt, T., Brown, G., Brown, M., Dabney, M., Wiley, O., & Weddington, G. (2003). *The Assessment of African American Children.* California Speech-Language and Hearing Association Task Force.

CHAPTER 7

Healing Noose Scars: *Cultural Empathy and Corrective Emotional Experiences*

Adopting frameworks of multiple perspectives across disciplines is one of the most critical factors to effectively move the needle of wellness for Black men and boys. Much of the damage that riddles their ecology has come as a result of a monolithic view that has efficiently painted a picture inappropriately applied to all people. "… (W)e can note that just as most fourteenth century scientists found it difficult to cease viewing the earth as the center of the physical universe, so too do many of today's (behavioral) scientists find it difficult to cease viewing the Caucasian race or European culture as the center of the social universe" (X, McGee, Nobes, & X, 1975).

White collusion is described as acts driven by a conscious and/or unconscious need to maintain or gain group power. According to *Mindful of Race* author Ruth King, there are three common ways that Whites collude as they determine the level of allyship they will display. This is taken as a cost benefit analysis as to how much they would be willing to go against the single perspective operationalized in the White group norm. To avoid what King refers to as the "edginess", people employ the following strategies: the blindness of not seeing race, the insularity of sameness or the safety of silence (King, 2016).

In *American Slavery As It Is* (Weld, 1839), witnesses to the atrocities of enslavement share their eyewitness accounts. Whether these individuals were frozen bystanders, horrified spectators and/or complicit co-orchestrators, there were generations of White people who bore

© The Author(s) 2019   221
D. E. Grant Jr., *Black Men, Intergenerational Colonialism, and Behavioral Health*, https://doi.org/10.1007/978-3-030-21114-1_7

witness to the carnage of enslavement and all that was associated with it. One White witness recounted his story:

> When the slaves are whipped, either in public or private, they have their hands fastened by the wrists, with a rope or cord prepared for the purpose: this being thrown over beam, a limb of a tree, or something else, the culprit is drawn up and stretched by the arms as high as possible, without raising his feet from the ground or floor: and sometimes made to stand on tip-toe ... Wile under the lash, the bleeding victim writhes in agony, convulsed with torture. Thirty-nine lashes on the bare back, which tear the skin at almost every stroke, is what the South calls a very moderate punishment ... they sometimes leave them tied for hours together, bleeding at every wound. (Weld, 1839 p. 20)

In order to create safe spaces for Black men and boys, White people have to stop avoiding the "edginess" operationalized by deliberate color-blindness, isolationist's behaviors of homogeneous groups and the silence of hoping that it will cease to exist if not spoken aloud. Norman Lear and Bud Yorkin were prominent television producing and writing partners in the late 1950s. Their shows would run well into the late twentieth century with many of them being watched by younger contemporary generations of youth whose parents were children when these shows first aired. The duo was originally famous for hit sit-coms like Maude and All in the Family that circled around White families and central characters. They also employed a multiple perspectives lens that was evident in both of these shows. Either they were business men who capitalized on an untapped television market prime for advertisers or authentically interested in giving voice to a community often neglected unheard, or perhaps a bit of both. Good Times was a spin-off of Maude and featured a Black family that included an employed father, a mother who was a homemaker and three children who were not in gangs, using drugs or teen parents. The father, James Evans, played by actor John Amos was a strong, proud Black man who consistently faced the ills of American racism as a husband, a father, a worker and a citizen. The Evans family lived in a Chicago housing project, and the story line focused on the strength and resilience of a family faced with the daily reality of life where poverty and Blackness met. Good Times aired from 1974 to 1979 and was one of the only shows on television at the time that portrayed a fully assembled Black family. The team also brought Sanford & Son to television audiences. Sanford & Son, starring Redd Foxx, aired from 1972 to 1977. Set in the Los Angeles neighborhood of Watts, Foxx plays Fred G. Sanford, a widowed junk dealer. What is most interesting about the pair is that although they had a lens of multiple perspectives, one of their perspectives was grounded in a single story … until it wasn't (Democracy Now, 2016).

In an interview with Democracy Now (2016), Lear discusses when he was compelled to give one of his perspectives an additional story. In his interview, he describes how leaders from the Black Panther Party visited him to state their displeasure with the television portrayal of Black men that he was promoting. Their concern was that Black men had many stories and that the only Black man on TV with a family was one who had to work several jobs just to meet the top of the poverty's bottom rung. Lear decided that George Jefferson would now "move on up" from the Bunker's neighborhood on All in the Family to a "deluxe apartment in the sky" as the hit television's opening theme song goes. George Jefferson, played by Sherman Hemsley, and Louise, his wife, played by Isabel Sanford, were an upwardly mobile couple who gained wealth in the dry-cleaning business. For the first time on television, there was an unapologetically Black Black man on television … even more important was that his Blackness was neither weaponized nor punished. Louise volunteered at The Help Center with her best friend and neighbor Helen who was in an interracial marriage with a White man, Tom. The Jeffersons lived in a luxurious high rise, had a house keeper and a doorman. Black families like this did exist in real life but were never portrayed on television. America's next visualization of this would be a decade later when we met the Huxtables in 1984. They were a Brooklyn family where the mom, Claire, played by Phylicia Rashad, was an attorney and the dad Cliff, played by Bill Cosby, was a physician. Together they raised their five children in a Brooklyn Heights brownstone surrounded by Black art, jazz, HBCUs and cultural strength. The show ranked number one for five of its seven seasons. There were many young Blacks transitioning from their socio-economic positions of origin who used the Huxtables as a model by which to raise their children and situate the lives they were entering for which many had no real-life model. During the years the world got to know the Huxtable family crack cocaine was ravishing inner-city communities and children were being exposed to community dangers they had never seen. During these same years and the years following, aligned with the Cosby Show spin-off, *A Different World* which followed one Huxtable daughter to college, HBCU enrollment increased and support for these institutions thrived while other Black students found their ways to PWIs they may have never accessed (Whatley Matabane, & Merrritt, 2014).

Certainly one can find stereotypical flaws associated with each of these shows. Some might attribute them to signs of the times or the deliberate and effective satirical lenses through which these shows were created and filmed. To whatever we attribute those flaws, what is important to note is the reward for diversifying a perspective. Television, movie and streaming producers and directors could certainly continue telling the same story of Black men over and over or they could give a young Black director like Ryan Coogler $200 million to bring a non-colonialized, futuristic portrait of Africa to life. Black Panthers' all-star cast gave Black boys—for the first time ever—the message that they too were superheroes. The world came out to experience Wakanda and its ruler King T'Challa, played by HBCU graduate Chadwick Boseman. Coogler showed the film industry how diversifying a lens and opening the door to another perspective might bring about reward. Black Panther made over $1.35 billion worldwide (IMDb).

Contextualizing Development

Black babies of all socio-economic statuses born into Euronormative nations are immediately faced with the toxins of a racialized world resulting from the promulgation and wide acceptance of one single perspective, that of White male dominance. By toddlerhood and pre-school, they are immersed in environments where stereotypes influence and inform inter-actions and engagements with peers, caregivers and other adults, often-times occurring beyond conscious awareness to the actor or the observer. Because toddlers and pre-schoolers are at the start of Piaget's "Preoperational Stage" of development, adults believe that they lack the cognitive sophistication to understand hierarchical racial cues. Yale University's Child Study Center (Gilliam, Maupin, Reyes, Accavitti, & Shic, 2016) indicated that Black pre-schoolers in America are 3.6 times more likely to be punished by means of out of school suspension when compared to their three- and four-year-old White pre-school peers. The researchers further indicated that Black children make up 19% of pre-schoolers but represent 47% of the pre-schoolers suspended at least one time during the year (Gilliam et al., 2016).

Given such disparities at this early entry point in academia, it is hard to believe that adults continue to minimize a child's awareness of impropriety and disproportionality in this setting. Although minimized throughout literature and research, Black boys are provided with consistent messages related to their implicit and explicit inferiority, danger and dispensability. In fact, Dr. Walter Gilliam, primary researcher in the study above, cited the "Three B's" as the primary risk factors for school expulsion as "big, Black or boy" (Dreher, 2017). Whether these children come from homes where their cultural heritage is championed and celebrated or ignored and vilified, the ecological stimuli of exclusion, omission and expulsion create visceral experiences that jar and scar Black male babies and children.

In the context of cognitive development, these experiences can render young children tasked with managing a default identity schema grounded in an inferior behavioral framework, historically referred to as "playing the role of Negro" (Van Ausdale & Feagin, 2001 p. 35). Consistently being forced to play the inferior role while being exposed to tangibly damaging provocations will alter a child's schema for self-identity and self-esteem. The comparative number of Black action figures and superheroes, scarcity of Black central characters in story books and science fiction and consistent promotion of stereotypical images of Black men and boys in youth television programming work together to solidify an image and definition of self. In the study "The First R of Racism", using observations of preschool children, the authors recount scenario after scenario of three- and four-year olds operationalizing their learned racial identity roles. White children manifested privilege—using racial epithets, telling Black children what they could and could not do and resituating themselves in rooms to avoid contact with Black children—that had been both explicitly and implicitly provided to them. Black children occupied the inferior role, often seeking assistance from adults to remedy the injury provided by their opposite raced pre-school peers (Van Ausdale & Feagin, 2001).

"The ethics and pragmatics of individual and collective healing, restitution, resilience and recovery can be understood in terms of the self-vindicating loops between politics, structural violence, public discourse and embodied experience" (Kirmayer, Gone, & Moses, 2014, p. 1). The relationship between communities of color and behavioral health professionals has been historically tenuous at best, outright exploitative at worst. There are a variety of reasons why many of which have been explored throughout this study. Although there exists an array of behavioral health paradigms identified as culturally empathic to the needs of Black communities in general and Black men specifically, not all take a holistic look at both the incremental and collective impacts of ecological and existential factors at different stages across development for Black men and boys.

A myriad of events and activities mark the stages of development for all people born genetically male no matter their ethnic tradition or country of origin. Brain and motor development during early childhood and emotional and moral development in late childhood are all influenced and informed by each child's biology and the space in which this development occurs. The hormonal changes of puberty and sexual maturation of adolescence are not unique to Black boys but—like with other boys—the socio-cultural space in which they occur creates a unique experience for each group. Not only is adolescent development across all its domains—cognitive, physical, psycho-social, emotional and so on—impacted by the environment, it is also dependent upon the previous developmental stages, starting at conception with pre-natal considerations.

In 1967, The Plowden Committee report indicated that experienced primary school teachers in Great Britain failed to attribute the cause of any youth difficulty to "skin colour prejudice" (Dearden, 1968). This common perspective has held different iterations throughout history and in many ways rings true today, where countries like France refuse to even identify race as a quantitative variable in outcomes for its citizens. French psychologist Jean Piaget is responsible for one of the most contemporarily influential theoretical frameworks of cognitive development. Piaget's theory describes individuals as active participants in their learning who develop "schemas" as basic building blocks of knowledge and information used to organize past experiences as a sort of road map for future ones. These malleable schemas are reformed and transformed by the complementary processes of assimilation and accommodation. Individuals often minimize the scope of influence that early experiences in childhood and adolescence have on their foundational cognitive framework. Due in part to Piagetian theory, adults have a tough time conceiving that children can act on insight beyond the developmental stage in which they exist. This includes fundamental understandings of racial hierarchies prevalent in nations around the world.

We pay close attention to explicit trauma and adverse childhood experiences. We track how they influence behavioral health but often forget that the most noted model of cognitive development is grounded in the individual's proclivity to use early experiences to understand most all future ones. The cognitive developmental process of assimilation works with existing schemas to see how new objects and experiences fit into them. If the actor determines that the new experience fails to fit into any of their pre-existing schemas, they alter them or create new ones through the process of accommodation.

There has been significant attention paid to the lack of cultural empathy imbued in the most popularly used theories of development. Some argue that the linearity of the models, their grounding in individualistic contexts and the restrictive chronological age boundaries often work to patholo-gize non-dominant, collectivistic cultures. Taking into considerations those critiques, the developmental models of Piaget (cognitive), Kohlberg (moral), Erickson (psychosocial) and/or Freud (psychosexual) all con-tinue to inform critical benchmarks of development for all youth, even youth of non-dominant cultural, ethnic or racial backgrounds. In each of these stage models of development, the experiences that young children have as their chronology ushers them closer and closer to adolescence are critical to their navigation skills.

The primary goal of adolescent psychosocial development according to Erikson's model is identity achievement. As teens explore and re-evaluate the goals, worldviews and value systems passed down by their caregivers and community members, they find themselves on a journey of self-exploration. They will reject some, accept others and try on some new ones. Canadian psychologist, James Marcia, expanded the work of Erikson with a primary focus on adolescent development.

Table 7.1 illustrates Marcia's four stages (Meeus, 2018).

Table 7.1 Marcia's stages of psychosocial development contextualized (Meeus, 2018)

Stage	Characteristics	Contextualized
Diffusion	Adolescent fails to meaningfully explore goals, values or beliefs. The adolescent may not conceptualize an identity until they experience a crisis	Crises of racial animus could result in identity adoption grounded in dependency, insecurity and/or self-hate
Foreclosure	Adolescent commits prematurely before adequate exploration has provided enough information for a sound commitment	Historical trauma might result in caregivers passing an identity to the adolescent that they take on. They may later resent the identity
Moratorium	Adolescent actively explores goals, values and beliefs but is not compelled to commit	Adaptive personality characteristics can result if adolescents are provided with adequate details regarding identity options and a safe space in which to explore them
Achievement	Adolescent makes stable commitment based on sufficient exploration and details of varied identities	Healthy adaptive personality with high self-esteem and autonomy can result when the adolescent is provided with positive images across all identity options and groups

To truly account for the multiplicity of factors that contribute to outcomes for Black boys and men, an innovative approach to education across the lifespan must be adopted. This must happen in two very deliberate ways in nations across the globe. First, we need to improve mental wellness and trauma-informed education and curriculum for credentialed teachers across all domains of academia related to socio-emotional learning and enrichment. Secondly, we need to strategically enrich the protective factors for Black boys in academic settings from elementary to college. The following details specific and measurable ways in which teams of professionals, stakeholders and educators might be able to achieve these goals.

The first way schools help to improve outcomes for Black boys and men is to enhance the safety of the psycho-social elementary and high school classrooms for everyone. Most schools and districts implement socio-emotional learning curricula in silos absent a cohesive partnership with other stakeholders, particularly teachers. Educators are idyllically placed to see early warning signs of mental stress and other socio-cultural risk factors. Research suggests that most educators are "ill-prepared for this role, are not comfortable using psychiatric language and do not work well with non-teaching support staff in a multi-agency context" (Bostock, 2011). It has become increasingly clear that mental health education is not sufficiently represented in the course work for the credentialing of America's teachers. With appropriate training, academic professionals could be key players in preventative efforts that reduce risk factors and bolster protective factors related to school aged youth and their experience with stress, oppression and marginalization. California's Student Mental Health Policy Workgroup (SMHPW) has determined several factors that are believed to "strengthen and improve student mental wellness" (Clark, 2013). The following key competencies are identified gaps in credentialed teacher preparation that the researchers found:

- The ability to recognize and understand key signs of mental health conditions.
- The ability to understand the function and efficacy of available programs and services.
- The ability to employ knowledge and training that reduce the stigma of mental health.
- The ability to develop strategic skills to help students with mental health concerns succeed in the classroom.

Educators play a crucial role on the front lines of youth developmental health. When teachers are informed and confident in their knowledge and skills as it relates to mental health wellness, they are better able to bolster the protective factors and minimize the risk factors associated with healthy, pro-social psychic development and foster resilience when prevention is improbable. Studies on resilience suggest that positive early intervention and prevention strategies that focus on child–adult relationship quality, self-concept and self-control in young children may support mental health resilience to adversity (Durlak et al., 2011; Miller-Lewis, Searle, Sawyer, Baghurst, & Hedley, 2013).

One major mental health approach in which teachers can competently engage when properly trained is referenced as "competence enhancement". Competence enhancement addresses an individuals' ability to respond effectively to the many life challenges they confront (Miller-Lewis et al., 2013). When combined with an understanding of the effects of mental health, competence enhancement can be a very useful classroom tool. These efforts can be post-hoc in the form of early childhood mental health consultations (ECMHC) for teachers already in the classroom in addition to their inclusion as part of a state's teachers credentialing requirements.

The second set of efforts to strategically enrich the protective factors for Black boys in academic settings from elementary school through college is no easy feat given the history of academic disenfranchisement that has painted their experiences. There are five factors that when effectively implemented in a parallel but coordinated effort have the potential to synergize a sustainable system's shift for Black men and boys. When one accounts for the risk factors explored in this study and beyond, a multi-modal approach is required for success. Success of Black men and boys can be exponentially improved by:

- Increasing the numbers of Black male teachers in elementary education.
- Implementing anti-bias education across all curriculums.
- Enhancing support for and research on HBCUs.
- Providing Predominately White Institutions (PWIs) with tools, research and resources to support Black male achievement and degree completion.
- Expanding resources for professional and trade pathways with apprenticeship and job placement opportunities

Black men make up only 2% of the entire population of public school teachers in America. In addition, they are five times more likely to leave the profession than any other ethno-gender groups (Teach for America, 2018). This number is far more dismal for other Euronormative nations. Why is this important you ask? A 2017 study looked at longitudinal data from all public schools in North Carolina and found that Black students who had a Black male teacher in third, fourth or fifth grade were less likely to drop out of high school and more likely to hold college aspirations. The high school drop-out effect was seen most influentially among Black boys who experienced persistent poverty during the elementary school years. With one Black teacher in those critical developmental years, researchers demonstrated a reduction in school attrition probability of 39% and an increase of college aspirations by 29% for Black boys. It is further demonstrated that this effect is not acute. The active ingredient of exposure to Black male educators appears to hold a longevity of educational investment over time (Gershenson, Hart, Lindsay, & Papageorge, 2017).

Organizations like "Profound Gentleman", created by two Teach for America teachers in Charlotte, are aiming to operationalize solutions to the concerns unearthed in this research. Mario Jovan Shaw and Jason Terrell recognized the lack of numbers, cohesiveness and support for Black male teachers. They also recognized the critical value of Black men in the classroom for youth of all cultural traditions. According to their website, current and aspiring male educators of color are placed into regional cohorts led by an Impact Leader who serves as a life/career and instructional coach. They work with the coach to create an Impact Professional Development Plan where goals are established and an educational leadership pathway is developed around their "3C Focus areas": Character Development, Content Development and Community Impact (Teach for America, 2018). This program has already, in a short time, demonstrated a model of support and sustainability that will impact outcomes for Black children and should be used as a model for Black male teacher recruitment and retention. In one year, Profound Gentleman served 225 male educators of color who in turn worked with approximately 1800 boys of color (Teach for America, 2018).

Black children have been consistently injured by curriculum content. Gaping holes of omission and plain revisionist lies riddle the spirit and souls of Black boys throughout their entire academic experience. Louise Derman-Sparks, long time pre-school teacher at Perry Preschool Project and faculty member at Pacific Oaks College in Pasadena, CA, has worked for over 50 years on issues of diversity and social justice. She played a significant role in the development of the anti-bias curriculum, an activist approach to educational curricula which challenges racism, sexism, ableism and homophobia among other marginalizing thought paradigms. Derman-Sparks states that "(A)n anti-racist person is on a life-long journey that includes forming new understanding of and ways to live her or his racial identity and then increasing commitment to and engagement in anti-racism actions" (Derman-Sparks, Keenan, & Nimmo, 2015). Anti-Bias Education has four goals that all school curriculum development teams should aspire to achieve:

Table 7.2 summarizes the four goals of Anti-Bias Education Curriculum and provides contextualized outcomes associated with each goal.

Anti-bias education is an approach to teaching and learning designed to increase understanding of differences and their value to a respectful and civil society. It is positioned to actively challenge bias, stereotyping and all forms of discrimination in schools and communities. It incorporates inclusive curriculum that reflects diverse experiences and perspectives, instructional methods that advance all students' learning and strategies to create and sustain safe, inclusive and respectful learning communities (Derman-Sparks et al., 2015).

Table 7.2 Four goals of anti-bias education (Derman-Sparkes et al., 2015)

Goal	Contextualized
1 Each child will demonstrate self-awareness, confidence, family pride and positive social identities.	Supports outcomes connected to stage theories of development that rely upon positive early experiences to inform future identity explorations.
2 Each child will express comfort and joy with human diversity; accurate language for human differences; and deep, caring human connections.	Supports safe environments with a respectful lexicon to explore difference, decrease difference and enhance human intimacy and connectivity.
3 Each child will increasingly recognize unfairness, have language to describe unfairness and understand that unfairness hurts.	Creates an equity lens where children not only recognize injustice but have language to employ tools of allyship for marginalized classmates.
4 Each child will demonstrate empowerment and the skills to act, with others or alone, against prejudice and/or discrimination.	Children are empowered with a life-long tool box of advocacy tools that support healthy communities and outcomes for all groups.

Colleges and universities across the world prepare to accept Black male students each year. Although students gain entry into these institutions, the institutions themselves must engage in deliberate efforts to create environments where Black men not just enter into school but actually complete their degrees and gain access to career pathway tools. In America, college-bound Black men get to choose between PWIs and HBCUs. Black men from Canada, France and the UK have also attended American HBCUs, but schools with these designations don't exist in their countries.

HBCUs generate a nexus of pedagogy and tradition that links together research on racial identity development, critical race theory and Black student achievement. The reinforcement of shared cultural experiences, an understanding of racism's role on experiences with discrimination and opportunity access and the "socio-cognitive benefits of being exposed to highly educated Black people" all play a significant role in why HBCUs successfully graduate Black men at a high rate and why their alumni account for a high proportion of the small number of graduate degrees among Black men in America, all of whom are not African American (Toldson, 2018). Given the successes that HBCUs have seen with Black men, support for them should be deliberate, robust and include resources beyond just financial.

In order for colleges, PWIs specifically, to improve rates of retention and graduation for Black male college students, the following five factors must be attended to on each and every campus (Grant Jr., 2013):

1. Colleges and Universities must partner with under-resourced high schools. High schools that educate Black students often fail to offer college preparatory tracks, advance placement coursework, robust college counseling or seasoned educators. We must demand that our public schools offer the basic courses for college enrollment and success. Exposure to college and its benefits must begin in elementary school, particularly with Black boys (Toldson & Lewis, 2012). Additionally, we must demand that our schools employ seasoned educators and provide a technology-based education.

2. Colleges and universities must make creative environmental enhancements to support the matriculation needs of all students. High levels of institutional support, close contact with faculty mentors and campus activity involvement all positively impact success rates for Black male collegians. Some colleges have created programs that address these underlying student needs. Ohio State's Bell

National Resource Center (Bell National Resource Center), Georgia Board of Regent's African American Male Initiative (University System of Georgia), the Student African American Brotherhood (over 200 nationwide chapters) and the Institute for Higher Education Policy (Institute for Higher Education Policy) are just a few organizations and university based programs directly addressing the unique matriculation needs of Black men. These and other successful programs incorporate one-on-one mentoring, group meetings and workshops on personal development, leadership and professional development. Each of these organizations has demonstrated significant improvements in Black male graduation rates at their affiliated institutions and many more institutions should follow suit (Carnevale & Strohl, 2013; Grant Jr., 2013).

3. Educators must identify and filter out their preconceived notions and expectations of Black boys. Institutionalized racism has created inferior perceptions and expectations for Black men and boys. The Rosental Effect is a well-documented socio-psychological theory that proves how expectations impact performance and success across most all domains. The insidiousness of institutionalized racism makes it such that even Blacks adopt lowered expectations for their sons, brothers and nephews. Youth tend to subconsciously live up or down to the expectations set for them. When monolithic images of Black men and boys saturate our experiences, we begin to believe the hype. We must train parents and educators at all levels to identify the personal and professional factors that impact expectations and provide coaching to teachers on mindfulness practices, privilege and the dangers of low expectations. Books like Ruth King's *Mindful of Race; Transforming Race from the Inside Out* provides a great framework for educators to engage in the authentic work that makes them mindful of their privilege and potential injuries they might be responsible for if they don't increase self-awareness (Gross & Lo, 2018).

4. We must increase Black male access to top-tier universities. The dollars spent on students during their college matriculation directly correlate with improved graduation rates, increased access to graduate school and better economic outcomes in the job market. Top colleges and universities spend two-to-five times more money per student than less competitive schools and can afford to admit more students who require more financial assistance for matriculation than they currently serve. A Georgetown University study entitled

the *20% Solution* (Carnevale & Van der Werf, 2017) found huge disparities in enrollment demographics based on university type. White students were largely concentrated in the nation's 468 most selective and well-funded US colleges and universities while Black students found themselves disproportionately concentrated in more open access schools with lower funding. Black enrollment in top-tier universities has increased since the 1990s but that only tells half the story. Between 1995 and 2009, more than 80% of new White college students enrolled in one of the top 468 US colleges and universities. During this same period, more than seven out of ten Black and Latinx students went to the less competitive "open-access", two and four year colleges (Carnevale & Van der Werf, 2017). We must increase access to the nation's top tier universities for Black men if we want to avoid the separate and unequal fate that has befallen the nations K-12 education resulting in an academic and economic under class.

5. Colleges, universities and the US Department of Education must increase access to affordable tuition packages and improve student loan options. Educational costs are sky-rocketing and most families aren't able to independently finance a full four-year education. Many families have challenges justifying the accrual of tens of thousands of dollars in student loan debt, particularly low-income families. Increased availability of student loan forgiveness programs can curtail portions of educational costs for most all universities depending on the work setting chosen by the graduate. This does, however, require that matriculation costs be covered on the front end and that graduates spend a minimum number of years in a particular career role (Grant Jr., 2013).

These same activities result in more use of positive classroom management strategies (Conners-Burrow et al., 2013), all of which have correlations to protective factor enhancement. These and other types of coaching and teacher consultative actions can be integrated within existing mental health activities in schools and impact classroom effectiveness and child adaptation across multiple domains (Cappella et al., 2012).

There are a variety of approaches to fill the mental health training gaps identified in the current state of international teacher credentialing and training processes. Educators and mental health professionals must work together to develop, manage and implement a curriculum for masters' level education and administration students and current teachers that fluidly and effectively incorporate the factors necessary to create mindful awareness in school communities as it relates to their role in student wellness. All socio-emotional learning curricula must follow a strength-based, culturally competent approach grounded in result-driven research and mindfulness.

Ethno-Gender Stress

Existential racism is most often measured and assessed as race-related stress, perceived discrimination and racial trauma. The prevalence of these experiences as reported by Black people in Euronormative nations is remarkably high even when compared to other people of color in these same nations. Research across disciplines have associated these experiences with respondents' reports on perceived life satisfaction, well-being, overall distress, emotional reactivity and psychological symptomology, including but not limited to anxiety, anger, hyper-vigilance, avoidance, depression, low self-esteem and general distress (Carter et al., 2013). Due to the consistency, frequency and gravity of race-based experiences among Black people living in countries where the bar of normality is White and of European descent, it is hard to believe that more researchers have not yet sought to identify moderating factors of race-related stress and experiences with perceived discrimination.

For those researchers that have journeyed down this path, the attitudes associated with one's current ethnic identity status and the coping styles relied upon to manage experiences with racism and perceived discrimination have been highlighted as significant contributing variables to outcomes across several domains. Although highlighted, the aforementioned don't work to minimize research's attention to other, often less quantifiable, contributing variables. Personality characteristics, one's appraisal of the racism-related experience and the severity of the encounter all contribute to how individuals deal with the stressor, ultimately determining the level to which the psychological impact is mitigated or exacerbated.

Due to the ways in which Black men and boys have been and continue to be hyper-masculinized, some may also experience masculine discrepancy stress (MDS). Most all cultures around the world have a set of shared values and mores that dictate how boys and men should act. These gender roles provide an incentivized road map that reinforces behaviors, emotions, toys, games and engagement styles that are congruent with endorsed gender role. In many cases, men are "expected to be confident and asser-tive, hide vulnerable emotions and demonstrate fearlessness through risk-taking behavior, demonstrate sexual prowess and promiscuity, and establish dominance through aggression and violence" (Reidy, Smith-Darden, Vivolo-Kantor, Malone, & Kernsmith, 2018, p. 560). MDS is the stress created by a fear of not meeting these measurements of masculinity, whether by choice or ability.

Research indicated that youth who experience Gender Role Discrepancy (GRD) and the resulting MDS are more likely to be depressed, attempt suicide, abuse drugs and alcohol, initiate substance abuse before age 13, be sexually active, initiate sexual intercourse before age 13, report less satisfaction with life and endorse lower ratings of their overall psychologi-cal well-being (Reidy et al., 2018). Due to the environments that over sexualize Black women and hyper-masculinize Black men, the likelihood of a masculine definition predicated on a brutish stereotype is dispropor-tionately high. This forces Black boys into a space where they have to either live up to the false masculinity that has been created by others and presented to them by their trusted community models or run the risk of reprisal, isolation, bullying and punishment for following their internal locus of control that is consistently stifled as a result of incongruence with external models.

Both racial and gender identity are psychosocial factors known to influ-ence a variety of areas for all people living in heterogeneous nations, no matter how they might identify ethnically or where they sit along the non-binary continuum of gender identification. Although the risk factors of colorism in the unique ecologies of racially homogeneous nations—not to be confused with racially homogeneous communities within heteroge-neous nations—are important, the focus on interethnic oppression differs from that of intraracial oppression. Racial and gender identity development has been well-studied, and the various stage models that exist provide evidence into the nuances of our racialized societies and their unique arrangements. Understanding the models is certainly important but even more so might be the ways in which people manage the stress that results from the ecosystem's responses to their development.

Coping, for the purposes of this study, is defined as the tools, resources and strategies used to manage both the internal and external demands that threaten well-being or exceed anticipated resource allocation. Coping associated with race-related stress and perceived experiences with discrimi-nation is time and place based, varies with demands of the environment and others involved (children, peers, supervisees, parents, etc.) and is dependent upon both situational and dispositional factors. There are very few studies on the use of Africultural, Afrocentric or African Centered coping strategies to deal with racism-related stress. Although some of the most contemporary studies on acculturative-stress tackle this issue, researchers tend to intuitively focus on immigrant populations and their progeny as opposed to groups who have been native to a nation across generations.

The Africultural Coping Systems Inventory (ACSI) is a 30-item measure of culture-specific coping strategies employed by Black Americans in stressful situations. It was conceptualized in 2000 according to an African-centered philosophical framework. ACSI items were developed using informal interviews with African Americans, observations and a review of existing relevant literature. After several years of norming and exploratory factor analysis, the researchers identified a four-factor model to best represent culture-specific coping behaviors among African Americans: Cognitive/Emotional Debriefing, Spiritual-Centered Coping, Collective-Coping and Ritual Centered Coping. The Perceived Racism Scale (PRS) is another published measure aimed at assessing coping skill sets associated with racism. Although it has made noted contributions to the research in this domain, it has not garnered success in demonstrating meaningful insights regarding the manifestations of coping styles and strategies in relation to race-related stressors (Utsey, Adams, & Bolden, 2000).

Over a decade later, the Racism-Related Coping Scale (RRCS) was designed for similar reasons as the ACSI adding factors that address "resisting racism" noticeable absent from the earlier assessment inventory. The RRCS uses a 59-item inventory across which eight racism-related factors of coping have been identified. Endorsements of the factor-specific items access coping strategies and attitudes across a variety of lived racially based experiences.

Table 7.3 illustrates the eight factors identified in the RRCS and several identified responses individuals are asked to endorse as a part of the survey tool (Forsyth & Carter, 2014).

Because the utilization of effective resources to cope with racism-related encounters reduces individual stress responses by changing situational and dispositional appraisals from threats to challenges, it is imperative that researchers use this information to develop interventions that mitigate the "noxious psychological and physiological responses" to these inevitable stress-inducing encounters (Forsyth & Carter, 2014, p. 640). Research

Table 7.3 The eight factors identified in the RRCS and several identified responses individuals are asked to endorse as a part of the survey tool (Forsyth & Carter, 2014)

Factor loading	Racism-related coping scale item (Forsyth & Carter, pp. 637–638)
Racially conscious action	I worked to educate others about racismI made a conscious decision to try to patronize only Black-owned businesses and establishmentsI surrounded myself by people who can relate to my own experience
Empowered action	I took legal actionI told my story in a public forumI organized a group response
Constrained resistance	I only did the minimum to get by at my job as a form of resistanceI exaggerated behaviors that are perceived to be "Black" in order to intimidate people who are not in my racial groupI got revenge
Confrontation	I talked about it with the person(s) involved in order to express my feelingsI got into an angry verbal conflict with the person(s) involvedI confronted the person(s) involved and told them that their actions were racist
Hyper-vigilance	I decided that I could no longer trust White people (or people who are not Black)I thought constantly about why this happened to meI blamed myself for trusting people who are not Black
Bargaining	I tried to understand the perspective of the perpetratorI looked for an explanation other than racismI tried to convince myself that it wasn't that bad
Spiritual coping	I read a passage from the Bible (or other religious text) to give me strength/guidanceI prayed about itI tried to stay positive no matter what
Anger regulation	I fantasized about getting revengeI fantasized about harming the person(s) involved or damaging/destroying their propertyI reacted with humor or sarcasm, or mocked the person(s) involved

indicates that teaching coping flexibility promotes and reinforces self-efficacy (Schwartz & Rogers, 1994), a critical human characteristic whose existence is very much predicated upon experiences and biology (nature & nurture).

Researchers indicate that experiences with conditions like racism, poverty, emotional abuse and neglect often trigger traumatic stress responses and symptoms consistent with PTSD. As a result of trauma's narrow clinical definition, the capacity for the emotional pain at the core of these events to be acknowledged as traumatic is small (Carter, Muchow, & Pieterse, 2018). In most cases, even the most impactful encounters with daily racism and perceived discrimination don't rise to meet the DSM V criteria of exposure to actual or potential death, grave injury or sexual violence after directly experiencing or witnessing an event. This often results in a severe minimization of the dangers and ranges of experiences with racism that all people of color in Euronormative nations experience to differing degrees.

Race-Based Traumatic Stress Models apply the concept of traumatic stress to racial encounters and experiences. Using specific memories of racial encounters, the Race-Based Traumatic Stress Symptom Scale (RBTSSS) associates reactions to said encounters to specific emotional symptoms like: avoidance (people, situations, events), hyper-vigilance, intrusive thoughts, depression, anger, somatic symptoms and low self-esteem. The assessment further learns whether the recalled event was sudden, unexpected, out of their control and/or emotionally painful, characteristics aligned with the assessment of more traditionally recognized trauma stimuli.

Not unlike traditionally defined trauma experiences, racial encounters that threaten one's existential well-being, emotional sense of security and psychological groundedness come in many different forms.

> Racial threats ... can be subtle and systemic, intentional or unintentional, vague and ambiguous or direct and specific, acute or chronic and cumulative, and can be perpetrated by a person (individual racism), institutional policies and practices (institutional racism), or via cultural oppression and power (cultural racism). (Constantine & Sue, 2007, p. 632)

Researchers might better understand the mechanization of risk factors in racially injurious environments by studying more discrete racism-based constructs. Disaggregating racial injuries into categories like Complex Racism, Intergenerational/Historical Racism, Systems Induced Racism, Separation/Grief Racism, Vicarious Racism, Community Racism and Emotional Racism with similar levels of specificity utilized in the interdisciplinary fields of trauma studies will force the doors to a new dialogue open, one that attacks systems and not only individuals or organizations. Some researchers have identified experiences with and exposure to racism as an etiological variable implicit in the higher rates of PTSD among people of color consistently illustrated across trauma research (Carter et al., 2013).

Many families of African descent across the diaspora continue to value a collectivistic worldview. Many of these families are preserving this world-view in counter-contexts of Euronormative individualistic settings. Family-centered interventions have been shown to reduce internalizing symptoms and family conflict while improving family cohesion. Addressing core relational themes by enhancing communication, strengthening attachments and shaping familial interactions have been predictive of improvements in family functioning and adolescent health (Hogue, Dauber, Samuolis, & Liddle, 2006).

Clinicians must increase their awareness of the psychological impacts of intergenerational trauma on Black men and boys. Due to the relatively small population of Black mental health professionals, it is probable that Blacks are being served by clinicians who might phenotypically represent the exact systems that created the historic and contemporary traumas and injustices experienced by the youth and his ancestors or the elder and his children. One factor cited for the underutilization of mental health services by Blacks are attitudes of cultural mistrust toward White therapists. In this study, researchers looked at how perceived racial micro-aggressions in therapy with a Caucasian clinician impacted therapeutic alliance and ratings of counseling satisfaction, factors that both have direct, empirically driven causal relationships to outcomes (Constantine & Sue, 2007). Many will confuse this construct with the idea of ensuring that every Black client has a Black therapist. Please note this is not to be confused with "race-matching" where individuals believe that they can only be efficaciously served by a clinician who looks like them. Research has consistently debunked that rationale while still supporting a lack of diversity in the industry as an access issue.

"Racial micro-aggressions refer to subtle and commonplace exchanges that somehow convey insulting or demeaning messages to people of color … frequently result(ing) in the communication of denigrating messages" (Constantine & Sue, 2007, p. 143). It is necessary for clinicians, service providers and practitioners engaging in cross-cultural helping relationships with Black males to identify, monitor and address micro-aggressions within the context of each relationship. It is critical to successful relational engaging that professionals create models where they are consistently holding themselves accountable to the accumulation of tools that decrease their likelihood of micro-aggressing. One can never eliminate the chance for this to happen given the fact that bias will always exist in some capacity, but mindful awareness promotes safe environments, the ultimate goal.

Relational teaching occurs when educators and administrators acknowledge a student's whole life and works to create environments where they can engage more comfortably. Research demonstrates that when groups engage in relational learning tools, student learning and trust in the learning process improves (Hogue et al., 2006). Deliberate attention to this style of engagement between Black boys of all socio-economic statuses is critical to their success, particularly if they are struggling in school or are experiencing other stressors in their lives.

African-Centered—Africana, Afrocentric and Black—Psychology represents one of the foundational strength-based paradigms that honors the worldview of Black people, Black research and Black behavioral health. African-Centered Philosophy concerns itself with the processes and procedures that bring Pan-African ideology, pedagogy and theory into places where their influence on scholarly and philosophical research can be assessed. When combined, African-Centered Psychology and Philosophy create a synergy that could positively impact communities across the diaspora exponentially. Dr. Greg Carr—Africana Philosophy scholar—notes the value of historical continuity across disciplines to explicitly illustrate the development of African-centered theories across time and space.

Most intellectual intercourse on post-American Civil War race relations focused on issues of integration versus segregation. This philosophy was the underpinning for most all research and thought pieces of the time and even served to be highly influential in legislation and public policy. In "The Fire Next Time" (1963), James Baldwin—noted scholar, author and socio-cultural analyst—asked: "Do I really want to be integrated into a burning house?". Baldwin was born in Harlem, New York, in 1924. In 1948—at the age of 24—Baldwin moved to Paris, purportedly to escape American racism. He remained highly connected and involved in addressing the conditions of Black Americans in the USA while living in Southern France. He befriended some of the most notable Black American leaders and entertainers of his time: Dr. Martin Luther King Jr., Harry Belafonte, Josephine Baker, Malcolm X, Miles Davis, Nina Symone and Sidney Poitier were just a few of his contemporaries. Baldwin's international lens informed a view and paradigm that was reflective, immersive and geographically removed. Although he didn't live in the USA full time, America saw him as one of the most eloquent race and cultural critics. His articles were consistently published alongside his books, he was a regular presence at American Civil Rights activities and even met with US Senator Robert Kennedy to discuss civil rights legislation.

It is well known that enslaved Africans arrived to the Americas with different references for religion and spirituality. Depending on their land of origin and time of capture, they might have practiced Islam, Orisha and even Christianity. Nubians converted to Christianity in the sixth century but were soon converted by the Islamic movement, and Ethiopia was one of the only remaining Christian countries in sub-Saharan Africa. The

Yoruba language family are regionally of West Africa (Benin, Togo, Nigeria, Ghana and Sierra Leone), most of the places from where enslaved Africans were taken. The Orisha pantheon of gods incorporates the events that people experience and the spaces in which they occur. Although there are many Orisha, there are several that are found referenced more consistently than others in the oral Yoruba tradition: Olodumare (Sky Father/ Creator of world order), Eshu (Jokester/Trickster), Ogun (Giver of Iron/ Hunter and Warrior), Oranyiman (Fertility God), Olookun (Goddess of Oceans), Olosa (Goddess of lagoons), Shango (Thunder God), Oya (God of winds) and Orunmila (God of Wisdom). These gods and their powers traveled along with the enslaved across the Atlantic to the Caribbean, South America and North America. In many cases, these spiritual foundations were lost through both forced assimilation and coerced acculturation. There are however some existing Black communities that have maintained this connection to their continental ancestry.

The Gullah (Geechee) Nation on St. Helena Island in South Carolina has maintained traditions from the African continent in a way that few other communities of African descent in Euronormative nations have. The people of Gullah island live on the land that many of their ancestors were enslaved on. The islands along the coast of South Carolina were littered with plantations that were abandoned during the American Civil War. Land ownership by the enslaved population along the Sea Island, Hilton Head and St Helena grew. Gullah land owners purchased land during the Civil War which has been passed down in what became known as Heir's Property which is shared by a group of heirs to the property owners. Currently, these lands are being taken from these original heirs for development purposes, and much of this history might be lost (Vice News).

After emancipation, Blacks gained access to a more direct route to religion, particularly Christianity. Many African American leaders gained tools, skills and capacity as a result of their membership and/or participation in a Black religious organization, whether it was a mosque, a church or a Temple. Thousands of Blacks who played significant roles in the country's efforts at change, had foundations built from their role in a religious community. The skill set of each was honed by leadership roles (junior usher), presentations (holiday plays), accounting (mosque bookstore), fund raising (Sunday School bake sale), oration (youth conferences), community organizing (advocacy work) and event planning that were all a direct reflection of participation in the Black Church, Mosque or Temple. Black Baptist denominations allowed Blacks to preach while the others did not. Black denominations developed in many ways due to discrimination they experienced in the larger national Baptist system. The 1895 National Baptist Convention became the largest Black denomination in the country. With over 7.5 million members, it is today the largest African American organization in the country (Anderson, 2009). These churches, throughout history, have been the hubs of mobilization against enslavement, Jim Crow and the murders of Black people. Black churches in the UK and Canada often grew from a response to the racism and discrimination that Blacks felt in these countries when they attended White churches. Northern Black churches in America rose after the Great Migration.

The Nation of Islam (NOI) began in 1930 in Detroit, MI, as a construct that tied the Islamic religion to the socio-political condition of African Americans in the USA. Elijah Muhammed became NOI's leader in 1934, under whom Malcolm X rose to prominence in the 1950s. Some people describe the NOI as a divisive "Black supremacist" group, while others see it as a religious tradition that provided opportunities for true growth and development in Black communities across the country. In 1995, the NOI organized the Million Man March in Washington DC, a day of peace, solidarity and action for Black men across the world. It was a day where over one million Black men descended onto the National Mall to celebrate one another and renew their commitments to themselves, their communities and their families.

Black Liberation Theology was born in the 1960s when 51 Black pastors purchased a full-page ad in the New York Times to demand a more deliberate and aggressive approach to the fight against racism. The founder of Black Liberation Theology, Rev. James Cone, believes that the goal of Christianity is in fact one grounded in social justice and advocacy for those experiencing marginalization and disenfranchisement. Each of these spiritual frameworks can be and have been used to mobilize communities, enrich youth, develop leaders, rehearse musicians and train great orators. Today, we see Blacks adopting a wide array of religions and spiritual traditions. Buddhism, Hinduism and Atheism have become increasingly popular with Black people around the world.

Research demonstrates that membership in faith communities typically has benefits and provides protective factors across several domains of wellness. The strength of this benefit differs between studies (Rapoport & Ismond, 1996). "Orthodox religious beliefs and personal devotion have been identified as protective against suicide among Blacks. Participation in organized religious practices, such as church attendance, is linked to lower suicide risk in African Americans. Among Blacks with psychiatric disorders, religiosity has been found to delay age of onset of ideation as well as decrease the number of psychiatric disorders" (Barnes, 2016). It is important to note, juxtaposed to the protective factors of spirituality, that some Blacks have historically demonstrated an over-reliance on spiritual tools to the neglect of those tangible ones. One might pray that their diabetes will not result in an amputation, but if that prayer is not accompanied by behaviors, like insulin compliance, the outcomes become clear. Many religious orders have now adopted "health and wellness ministries" where professionals and peers support wellness systems in the community to promote resilience (Migdal & MacDonald, 2013).

Resiliency Theory provides people with opportunities to create programs, evaluate learning and assess wellness using a strength-based lens. It grew from studies on youth adversity when researchers began to explore the reasons why some youth grew to be healthy adults in spite of or because of the ecological risks they encountered. The theory focuses on "positive contextual, social, and individual variables that interfere or disrupt developmental trajectories" that, in many circumstances, results in problem behaviors, mental distress and poor health outcomes. Understanding the mechanisms by which resiliency factors counteract, protect against or inoculate youth from the maladaptive outcomes of the risks is key (Zimmerman, 2013).

Post-traumatic growth is a late twentieth-century outgrowth of resiliency theory. It is the "positive psychological change experienced as a result of the struggle with highly challenging life circumstances" (Tedeschi & Calhoun, 2004, p. 1). It tends to occur in five general areas:

- Opportunities that would not have emerged absent the struggle.
- Relationships that have changed in positive or self-preserving ways.
- New awareness and/or increase of one's strength
- A greater appreciation for life in general
- A deepened sense of spirituality

Each has the capacity to create corrective emotional experiences that allow men and boys to gain practical evidence of success to counter and dismantle the narratives of danger and pain (Collier, 2016). There are many factors that contribute to one's ability to "bounce back". Besides internal factors, communities must ensure that due diligence is dedicated to the minimization of racial trauma and stress. Efforts that exist to acknowledge and mitigate traumas when they do occur help to optimize resiliency opportunities.

Conclusion

When venturing on the journey to support positive outcomes for Black men, there are many factors that require one's attention. It is critical to honor both the connectedness and uniqueness of Black men and boys across the diaspora. There is value to the construction of a knowledge base that joins together the historic, geographic, chronosystemic and existential components of an ethno-gender group's experience. Although navigating and bridging each component is no simple task, practices of cultural humility require that individualized tools fill our boxes to optimize safety and security for all people.

Black men and boys around the world are saturated with rich traditions of family and food, a love for humanity, a strong desire to live their best lives within the context of both their geographic and experiential spaces and a desire to live free and happy, as defined and designed by them. These common threads shared through the human experience and across most all national traditions create a contextual connectedness among most all people. The ability to conceptualize these relationships and interactions through a global lens results in observations and associations often lost through country of origin centeredness and insularity. For many, a globalized understanding both brings attention to our common universal humanity and to the seething tension and anxiety associated with aspects of our collective humanity that are more common for some than others.

The Black Community hosts many strong and resilient qualities. The natural selection of those Africans who survived colonialism and the Middle Passage left a gene pool worth note. A group's legacy cannot be left to languish as a result of unseen, unaddressed and untended psychological, socio-cultural, medical and adjudicative injuries. The world must make an intentional and strategic shift, opening dialogue about the behavioral health and unique wellness needs of Black men and boys. Demands must be made that the psychological community offer culturally empathic services and train culturally humble clinicians. Families must acknowledge that Uncle Pete suffered from bipolar disorder, and that he did not just have a "nervous breakdown". Adjudicating bodies must see that Tariq suffered from PTSD and was not just an incorrigible kid on drugs.

Although difficult for the naked eye to see, systems of disparity across geographically separated groups of people with a common ethno-historical heritage in very specific ecological contexts become strikingly clear when presented cohesively. Eurocentric frameworks of normality across continents are dangerous to the well-being of Black males across the lifespan. Across the USA, France, Canada and the UK, citizens who happen to be male and of African descent exist at an intersectionality resulting in both the post-traumatic growth and the dire consequences described throughout this study. If we are serious about positively impacting suicide, fatherlessness, incarceration, hyper-masculinity, school attrition, community violence, generational poverty, substance abuse, misdiagnoses, underemployment and illiteracy among Black men and boys, we must act strategically with loving and compassionate urgency.

REFERENCES

Anderson, M. (2009). *National Baptist Convention*. Black Past. Retrieved from https://www.Blackpast.org/african-american-history/national-baptist-convention-usa-inc-1895/

Barnes, M. (2016). *Black Suicide Matters: Facts You Should Know*. Rolling Out. Retrieved from https://rollingout.com/2016/06/05/Black-suicide-matters-facts-you-should-know/

Bell National Resource Center on the African American Male. Retrieved from https://odi.osu.edu/bell-national-resource-center/

Bostock, J. (2011). Why Wait Until Qualified: The Benefits and Experiences of Undergoing Mental Health Awareness Training for PGCE Students. *Pastoral Care in Education, 29*(2), 103–115.

Cappella, E., Hamre, B. K., Kim, H. Y., Henry, D. B., Frazier, S. L., Atkins, M. S., et al. (2012). Teacher Consultation and Coaching Within Mental Health Practice: Classroom and Child Effects in Urban Elementary Schools. *Journal of Consulting & Clinical Psychology, 80*(4), 597–610.

Carnevale, A. P., & Strohl, J. (2013). *Separate and Unequal; How Higher Education Reinforces the Intergenerational Reproduction of White Racial Privilege*. Georgetown University. Retrieved from https://cew.georgetown.edu/wp-content/uploads/SeparateUnequal.FR_.pdf

Carnevale, A. P., & Van der Werf, M. (2017). *The 20% Solution; Selective Colleges Can Afford to Admit More Pell Grant Recipients*. Georgetown University. Retrieved from https://1gyhoq479ufd3yna29x7ubjn-wpengine.netdna-ssl.com/wp-content/uploads/The-20-Percent-Solution-web.pdf

Carter, R. T., Mazzula, S., Victoria, R., Vazquez, R., Hall, S., Smith, S., et al. (2013). Initial Development of the Race-Based Traumatic Stress Symptom

Scale: Assessing the Emotional Impact of Racism. *Psychological Trauma: Theory, Research, Practice, and Policy, 5*(1), 1–9. Retrieved form https://doi-org.lib.pepperdine.edu/10.1037/a0025911

Carter, R. T., Muchow, C., & Pieterse, A. L. (2018). Construct, Predictive Validity, and Measurement Equivalence of the Race-Based Traumatic Stress Symptom Scale for Black Americans. *Traumatology, 24*(1), 8–16.

Clark, W. (2013). *View Points: Teacher Credentialing Should Include Mental Health Training*. Sacramento Bee. Retrieved from http://www.sacbee.com/2013/07/31/5610226/teacher-credentialing-should-include.html

Collier, L. (2016). Growth After Trauma. *Monitor on Psychology, 47*(10), 48.

Conners-Burrow, N., McKelvey, L., Sockwell, L., Harman Ehrentraut, J., Adams, S., & Whiteside-Mansell, L. (2013). Beginning to "Unpack" the Infant Mental Health Consultation: Types of Consultation Services and Their Impact on Teachers. *Infant Mental Health Journal, 34*(4), 280–289.

Constantine, M. G., & Sue, D. W. (2007). Perceptions of Racial Microaggressions Among Black Supervisees in Cross-Racial Dyads. *Journal of Counseling Psychology, 54*(2), 142–153.

Dearden, R. F. (1968). *The Philosophy of Primary Education (RLE Edu K)*. London: Routledge.

Democracy Now. (2016). *TV Legend Norman Lear on Black Panthers, Nixon's Enemies List and What Gives Him Hope*. Retrieved from https://www.youtube.com/watch?v=oSwbnoCo8UQ

Derman-Sparks, L., Keenan, D., & Nimmo, J. (2015). *Leading Anti-Bias Early Childhood Programs: A Guide for Change*. Washington, DC: National Association for the Education of Young Children.

Dreher, A. (2017). *'Big, Black or Boy' Preschoolers Face Higher Expulsions and Suspensions*. Retrieved from http://www.jacksonfreepress.com/news/2017/mar/23/big-Black-or-boy-preschoolers-face-higher-expulsio/

Durlak, J. A., Weissberg, R. P., Dymnicki, A. B., Taylor, R. D., & Schellinger, K. B. (2011). The Impact of Enhancing Students' Social and Emotional Learning: A Meta-Analysis of School-Based Universal Interventions. *Child Development, 82*, 405–432.

Forsyth, J. M., & Carter, R. T. (2014). Development and Preliminary Validation of the Racism-Related Coping Scale. *Psychological Trauma: Theory, Research, Practice, and Policy, 6*(6), 632–643.

Gershenson, S., Hart, C., Lindsay, C., & Papageorge, N. (2017). *The Long-Run Impacts of Same-Race Teachers*. IZA Institute of Labor Economics. Retrieved from http://ftp.iza.org/dp10630.pdf

Gilliam, W., Maupin, A., Reyes, C., Accavitti, M., & Shic, F. (2016). *Do Early Educators' Implicit Biases Regarding Sex and Race Relate to Behavior Expectations and Recommendations of Pre-school Expulsions and Suspensions?* New Haven, CT: Yale University Child Study Center.

Grant, Jr., D. E. (2013). *Reversing the Black Male College Drop-Out Crisis*. Ebony Magazine. Retrieved from https://www.ebony.com/news/reversing-the-Black-male-college-drop-out-crisis-756/#axzz2gbVKGtUE

Gross, N., & Lo, C. (2018). Relational Teaching and Learning After Loss: Evidence from Black Adolescent Male Students and Their Teachers. *School Psychology Quarterly, 33*(3), 381–389.

Hogue, A., Dauber, S., Samuolis, J., & Liddle, H. A. (2006). Treatment Techniques and Outcomes in Multidimensional Family Therapy for Adolescent Behavior Problems. *Journal of Family Psychology, 20*(4), 535–543.

IMDb. Retrieved June 2019, from https://www.imdb.com/title/tt1825683/.

Institute for Higher Education Policy (IHEP). Retrieved from http://www.ihep.org/about-ihep

King, R. (2016). *Mindful of Race; Transforming Race from the Inside Out*. Boulder, CO: Soundstrue.

Kirmayer, L., Gone, J., & Moses, J. (2014). Rethinking Historical Trauma. *Transcultural Psychiatry, 51*(3), 299–319.

Meeus, W. (2018). The Identity Status Continuum Revisited: A Comparison of Longitudinal Findings with Marcia's Model and Dual Cycle Models. *European Psychologist, 23*(4), 289–299.

Migdal, L., & MacDonald, D. A. (2013). Clarifying the Relation Between Spirituality and Well-Being. *Journal of Nervous and Mental Disorders, 201*(4), 274–280.

Miller-Lewis, L., Searle, A. K., Sawyer, M. G., Baghurst, P. A., & Hedley, D. (2013). Resource Factors for Mental Health Resilience in Early Childhood. An Analysis with Multiple Methodologies. *Child & Adolescent Psychiatry & Mental Health, 7*(1), 1–23.

Rapoport, J., & Ismond, D. (1996). *DSM IV Training Guide for Diagnosis of Childhood Disorders*. New York: Brunner-Routledge.

Reidy, D. E., Smith-Darden, J. P., Vivolo-Kantor, A. M., Malone, C. A., & Kernsmith, P. D. (2018). Masculine Discrepancy Stress and Psychosocial Maladjustment: Implications for Behavioral and Mental Health of Adolescent Boys. *Psychology of Men & Masculinity, 19*(4), 560–569.

Schwartz, C. E., & Rogers, M. P. (1994). Designing a Psychosocial Intervention to Teach Coping Flexibility. *Rehabilitation Psychology, 39*(1), 57–72.

Student African American Brotherhood. Retrieved from http://saabnational.org/

Teach for America. (2018). *What It Takes to Retain Black Male Teachers*. Retrieved from https://www.teachforamerica.org/stories/what-it-takes-to-retain-Black-male-teachers

Tedeschi, R., & Calhoun, L. (2004). Posttraumatic Growth: Conceptual Foundations and Empirical Evidence. *Psychological Inquiry, 115*(1), 1–18.

Toldson, I. (2018). Why Historically Black Colleges and Universities Are Successful with Graduating Black Baccalaureat Students Who Subsequently Ear Doctorates in STEM (Editor's Comments). *The Journal of Negro Education, 87*(2), 95–98.

Toldson, I. A., & Lewis, C. W. (2012). *Challenge the Status Quo: Academic Success among School-Age African American Males*. Washington, DC: Congressional Black Caucus Foundation, Inc.

University System of Georgia. *African American Male Initiative*. Retrieved from https://www.usg.edu/aami/

Utsey, S. O., Adams, E. P., & Bolden, M. (2000). Development and Initial Validation of the Africultural Coping Systems Inventory. *Journal of Black Psychology, 26*(2), 194–215.

Van Ausdale, D., & Feagin, J. (2001). *The First R: How Children Learn Race and Racism*. Lanham, MD: Rowman & Littlefield Publishers Inc.

Vice News. *A Vanishing History: Gullah Geechee Nation*. Retrieved from https://www.youtube.com/watch?v=SqDTJogdWmA

Weld, D. T. (1839). *American Slavery as It Is: Testimony of a Thousand Witnesses*. Mineola, NY: Dover Publications.

Whatley Matabane, P., & Merrritt, B. (2014). Media Use, Gender, and African American College Attendance: The Cosby Show Effect. *Howard Journal of Communications, 25*(4), 452–471.

X (Clark), C., McGee, D. P., Nobles, W., X (Weems), L. (1975). Voodoo or IQ: An Introduction to African Psychology. *Journal of Black Psychology, 1*(2), 9–29.

Zimmerman, M. A. (2013). Resiliency Theory: A Strengths-Based Approach to Research and Practice for Adolescent Health. *Education & Behavior: The Official Publication of the Society for Public Health Education, 40*(4), 381–383.

INDEX

© The Author(s) 2019
D. E. Grant Jr., *Black Men, Intergenerational Colonialism, and
Behavioral Health*, https://doi.org/10.1007/978-3-030-21114-1